Kristi,
Keep pla... and
Good ...

Yohnn...

NUTRITION
A Word of Wisdom

NUTRITION
A Word of Wisdom

Dr. Scott A Johnson
Traditional Naturopath

Cover design and photos by Scott A. Johnson
Alluring Books Press. Orem, Utah.

IMPORTANT NOTICE

The purpose of this book is to educate. While every effort has been made to ensure accuracy, it is not intended to replace any medical advice or to halt proper medical treatment. Rather as information for the reader to utilize as he or she sees fit as part of a personal health and wellness plan. This book is sold with the understanding that the author shall have no liability for any injury or harm alleged to be caused directly or indirectly by its contents.

Contents

Introduction

We live in a world where convenience outweighs nutrition. We have been conditioned to believe that food must come in a box, can, or bag and that it must be easy and quick to prepare. We eat processed and empty calories as the bulk of our diet, because they are more convenient than making the effort to eat healthily. Moreover, we miss out on the experiences of socializing and interacting with our families as we cook and prepare meals. The result of this unhealthy diet is a significant increase in chronic illnesses and degenerative diseases. In fact, poor nutrition is a major contributing factor in the three leading causes of death among Americans: heart disease, cancer, and stroke.

Contrary to logic, the diets currently consumed in industrialized nations are inferior when compared to those consumed decades ago. In the past, only the wealthy could afford the luxury of unhealthy meals. Ironically, "unindustrialized" communities have lower levels of chronic illnesses and avoid the common diseases that are so prevalent in affluent societies. Poor nutritional habits slowly weaken our immune system and break down our resistance to diseases. This may take years to become apparent, but poor nutritional habits will eventually result in negative consequences.

There are virtually as many opinions regarding healthy food choices as there are people on the planet. So how do we determine what is a health promoting diet? The intent of this book is to provide nutritional guidance and to empower individuals to make correct dietary choices. Its guidance can benefit everyone, regardless of race, religion, or socioeconomic status. It is based upon a revelation, essentially a guide to nutrition, as given from God to His prophet Joseph Smith. Even though it is a revelation directed toward members of the Church of Jesus Christ of Latter Day Saints, it does not preclude people of all religious denominations from benefiting from its counsel.

The information is offered for the benefit of all, and not by constraint or force. In other words, you can take the advice or leave it. It is my desire and obligation to share my knowledge of health and nutrition and to educate and inform you of appropriate dietary measures. Then, I leave it to you to determine if these suggestions make sense for yourself and your family. It is my hope that all who read the contents of this book will receive knowledge beneficial to their health and the health of their families. Hopefully, the thoughts presented here will establish daily dietary habits that will promote the health of the body and the soul.

Unfortunately, we tend to focus on a small portion of the Word of Wisdom – the don'ts. This is despite the fact that the bulk of this revelation teaches us what we should eat. In order to live the Word of Wisdom to its fullest, we must incorporate the do's as well as avoid the don'ts. If you follow the wise counsel the Lord has given, you will achieve optimal health and wellness. Of course, this doesn't mean you will be disease or illness free, but it will mean that you will establish the greatest possible health for yourself as an individual. Moreover, you may decrease your health care expenses in the process.

An interesting article recently proclaimed that if no Americans were fat, the combined savings in health, food, clothing, and efficiencies would result in a savings of $4,270 per American, or $487 billion[1]. In the United States, more money is spent on healthcare than on education. If everyone followed the Lord's counsel, I am certain there would be less disease, less disability, and further enriched lives. We would live not just longer, but healthier, lives, with greater opportunity to share them to the fullest with those we love.

The counsel in this book is not meant to encourage extremism in diet, but to promote thoughtful deliberation of one's current nutritional practices and state of health. Moderation really is the key. It does take effort, but it is not difficult to incorporate. Besides, isn't your health worth it?

Principles of this revelation and the suggestions contained in this book are best taught when young, but can be incorporated at any age. The sooner a person learns proper nutritional habits, the earlier they can establish personal optimal health. My desire is that parents will learn better dietary habits from this book and will teach them to their children, thus enabling them to perpetuate good habits to the next generation and the next; breaking the current trend toward convenience at the expense of nutrition. Ultimately, I hope this will result in healthier generations, thus breaking the cycle of obesity, disease, and poor health currently being propagated by unhealthy dietary habits and choices.

I possess a personal witness of the divinity and importance of this revelation. I have seen its benefits in my own life, and in the lives of others. President Gordon B. Hinckley said, "The code of health followed by the Latter-day Saints, which is so widely praised in these days of cancer and heart research, is in reality a revelation given to Joseph Smith in 1833 as a 'Word of Wisdom' from the Lord (see D&C 89:1). In no conceivable way could it have come of the dietary literature of the time, nor from the mind of the man who announced it. Today, in terms of medical research, it is a miracle whose observance has saved incalculable suffering and premature death for uncounted tens of thousands[2]." To his testimony I add mine, that the Word of Wisdom is a revelation from God, the observance of which will prevent unnecessary suffering and death, and enhance the health of all who endeavor to live it to its fullest.

Chapter 1

Doctrine & Covenants 89:1-4

"A WORD OF WISDOM, for the benefit of the council of high priests, assembled in Kirtland, and the church, and also the saints in Zion—

To be sent greeting; not by commandment or constraint, but by revelation and the word of wisdom, showing forth the order and will of God in the temporal salvation of the saints in the last days—

Given for a principle with promise, adapted to the capacity of the weak and the weakest of all saints, who are or can be called saints.

Behold, verily, thus saith the Lord unto you: In consequence of evils and designs which do and will exist in the hearts of conspiring men in the last days, I have warned you, and forewarn you, by giving unto you this word of wisdom by revelation-"

Nutrition is an enormous and controversial subject. The information that can be found regarding this subject is vast, and the number of experts in the field of nutrition is equally daunting. Although numerous books purport to contain the best diet for your health, in fact there is not one ideal diet but many, each based on the specific needs and circumstances of a particular individual. We are all metabolically different and require different nutrients. There are numerous fad diets, each claiming to be the best for weight loss, but they all approach this concept in different and often contradictory ways. If you perform an Internet search for nutritional subjects, you will get an enormous number of people and webs sites, all willing to share "expert" advice. Much of this advice is based on the fact that they are trying to sell you a product.

Healthy eating is challenging and it takes effort, but it is vital and plays the most critical role in maintaining our health. Nutrition truly is the foundation of our health. "You are what you eat" is more literal than some of us would like to believe. What we eat eventually enters and makes up the content of our blood stream. Our food is utilized as the building blocks of our body. Proper nourishment is necessary for cells to rebuild and function properly.

Nutrition is particularly important for the growth and development of children and adolescents, but remains important for all ages in order to reduce the risk of chronic illnesses.

According to the American Institute for Cancer Research, thirty to forty percent of cancers are nutrition-related.[3] If we were to alter our diets to include healthier and more nutritious choices, how many of the 553,888[4] cancer deaths per year could be avoided?

There are many diseases and conditions associated with poor nutrition, including cardiovascular disease, stroke, diabetes, osteoporosis, and obesity. According to one study, about sixteen percent of mortality in men and nine percent in women could be eliminated by appropriate nutritional behaviors.[5] This is a conservative number in my opinion. I believe that most disease results from poor nutrition, which provides the perfect environment for disease to flourish. Many foreign and disease causing invaders will only thrive and cause illness if they are provided the right environment and if the host's immune system is not strong enough to fight them off. How many deaths could be avoided with a few small changes in dietary habits? The answer is a significant number. Not to mention the improved quality of life that would be achieved.

Yes, Americans are living longer than ever before – but what quality of life are we enjoying? We, in fact, are not living healthier, better quality lives. This is obvious as we see our nursing homes full of sick, decrepit, and crippled elderly. Quantity does not always equal quality! We have come to accept certain illnesses and conditions as a normal part of aging, when this is not actually the truth. Many of these conditions and illnesses are present based on poor dietary and lifestyle choices.

Some would say that it is too expensive to eat healthy meals. In the short term, it certainly is more expensive to purchase healthy products versus products devoid of proper and essential nutrients. However, can you really put a price tag on your health? How much is your good health worth? In the long term, healthy eating and providing your body with proper nutrition will save you untold dollars in health care costs and lost wages.

The authors of *The China Study* state that "eating the right way would largely obviate the enormous costs of using drugs, as well as their side effects. Fewer people would need to wage lengthy, expensive battles with chronic disease in hospitals over their last years of life. Health care costs would drop and medical mistakes would wane as premature death plummeted. In essence, our health care system would finally protect and promote our health as it is meant to do."[6] You can pay a little more now for healthy eating or pay a lot later in health care expenses.

Another question may be the genetics factor. This is, of course, a determining factor in disease; but, much as a light switch has the capability to provide light, it cannot do so without an external factor. In other words, our bodies may have a genetic predisposition to a disease or condition but will not manifest this condition unless an internal switch is turned on. This internal switch is often poor nutrition. The more substandard our nutrition is, the greater will be the possibility of turning on those genetic switches.

A gardener will tell you that a seed is no good unless you can provide the proper soil, nutrients, water, and sunlight required for that seed to mature and develop into a plant. Theoretically, if we were to keep our bodies healthy enough, we would not allow the disease (seed) the proper nutrients or environment (soil) to develop. Proper dietary habits provide proper nutrients for optimal functioning of the immune system and a less hospitable environment for disease to develop.

Nutrition plays a crucial role in our immune system. The immune system is a complex system of specialized cells and organs that work together to prevent invasion by foreign substances and to remove foreign and harmful invaders if they do invade the body. In our bodies, there are two classes of specialized cells called lymphocytes: the B cells, which circulate in the blood locating and marking antigens (foreign invaders) for destruction; and the T cells, which also patrol for invaders but in addition play a role in the actual removal and destruction of the antigens.

Poor nutrition primarily affects the alarm portion of the immune system – the part that notifies the body of foreign invaders and marks them for destruction. This alarm failure allows these antigens to progress freely through the body undetected. This is similar to having an alarm system in your home without any power supplied to the alarm unit. Eventually, disease or illness will result. Nutrient deficiencies can also suppress the immune system, allowing the invaders more activity and opportunity to cause damage, disease, or illness. Proper nutrition is the body's best defense against foreign invaders because it supports optimal immune system function.

In the United States today, one epidemic disease that can be attributed to poor dietary habits is obesity. The more extra weight an individual carries, the greater is the risk for any number of chronic diseases. Being overweight increases your risk of diabetes, arthritis, osteoarthritis, high blood pressure, and cardiovascular disease. Obesity can also be emotionally taxing, as it devastates a person's self-esteem and confidence. This lack of confidence in physical appearance may in turn drive the obese person to avoid society and interactions with others. Thus, the obese may inadvertently shut out the help and assistance that they need in order to start out on the path to better health.

It seems that there is a new miracle weight loss pill, surgery, or plan introduced every day. Surgeons modify the stomach, making it as small as a thumb; others promote harmful drugs; and yet others encourage dangerous diets or lifestyle factors, all in the name of losing weight. Unscrupulous people take the money of overweight and obese persons, and in turn provide little more than the false hope that their miracle "cure" will result in weight loss. There are innumerable weight loss programs and diets; some are backed by doctors or other experts in the field of nutrition. Some diets advocate high-protein, low-carbohydrate consumption, when in fact the healthiest diet you can consume is one high in carbohydrates. The important factor is the type of carbohydrates that you consume. Refined sugar and white flour are so called "empty calories" that will cause weight gain. The bottom line is that a healthy and proper diet, combined with moderate exercise, is the best way to maintain a healthy weight. We simply can't continue to sit in front of the television or computer for hours at a time, snacking on junk food, and expect to maintain a healthy weight.

Chronic illnesses and degenerative diseases are no longer plagues that only affect the elderly. More and more, our children and very young adults are succumbing to life altering and crippling illnesses. Diseases that used to be considered adult diseases are now increasingly more common among children, including high blood pressure, asthma, and diabetes. All of these diseases can place limitations on the activities of these children, resulting in an inferior quality of life. The incidence of childhood asthma has increased approximately two-hundred forty-seven percent in the last twenty-five years.[7] Two studies have concluded that type 1 diabetes (a chronic condition where the pancreas does not produce enough insulin to properly control blood sugar) has not only increased significantly, but now strikes children at a younger age.[89] It is tragic to watch children suffer with such horrible and debilitating diseases. We, as parents, need to make a more concerted effort to provide the proper type of nutrition to our children that affords them the best chance to avoid these types of diseases.

If you ask five nutritionists for an opinion on a particular nutrient, you are likely to receive five different views. There are often contradictory studies and scientific publications regarding the same nutrient. Look at the butter/margarine debate, for example. One study will assert that margarine is healthier, while another asserts butter is better, with both sides of the debate presenting "scientific" data to back up their claims. What can you believe when contradictory studies exist?

These studies are often biased, depending on who is funding the study. For example, one study funded by the corporate parent of Lipton tea suggested that up to forty ounces of unsweetened coffee or tea and twelve ounces of beer daily is healthy.[10] This study asserted that unsweetened tea and coffee are acceptable substitutes for water. It is quite comical to believe that a study funded and initiated by Lipton would produce any other results than they did. The person conducting the study obviously had a vested interest in ascertaining this conclusion.

Data may be interpreted favorably or unfavorably, based on the views and or beliefs of the individual conducting the study. If a scientist has a particular view about a nutrient, it is human nature to hope for favorable results for that nutrient. The scientist will do everything possible to prove his or her hypothesis or belief to be correct. Bias frequently sneaks into studies and articles, probably more than we know. In fact, an article published in PLoS Medicine, a peer reviewed journal, concluded that food industry funding of nutrition-related scientific articles may bias the articles in preference toward the sponsor's products, with substantial implications for public health.[11] This article found that eighty-seven percent of studies funded by industry had results favorable or neutral to the industry, while only sixty-one percent of non-industry funded studies were favorable or neutral to the industry. This is a significant difference and demonstrates the bias inherent to industry-funded studies. It is the equivalent of Ford Motor Company requesting and paying for a study to determine if their vehicles are reliable. The results of these studies are obviously frequently manipulated and interpreted sympathetically toward the sponsor, or the desired outcome of the individual conducting the study. When a new study is released, touting a benefit or consequence of a product, it would be prudent to investigate the funding of the study, as well as the background of the person or persons who conducted the study.

With this much information to sort through and with contradictory scientific studies commonplace, are we then doomed to never have accurate and unbiased information about nutrition? The answer to that question is no. Is there a better source than God when it comes to nutrition? He is the designer and creator of our bodies and knows what is best for them. He is the master nutritionist, chemist, and biologist. In contrast to the philosophies of men and the scientific community, God is never changing – He remains constant and unvarying. He wants His children to be healthy and has given us a blueprint of what constitutes proper and healthful nutrition in the Word of Wisdom. Given the complexity of the human organism, who better to consult about nutrition than our Creator?

He will not force the Word of Wisdom on any of his children, but it is His will that we are healthy and have the knowledge available to take care of our bodies. God has offered us some of His wisdom and knowledge of nutrition and the human body and we may choose to accept or reject that information. Not only does He offer us this knowledge, He provides us a promise that we will have optimal health, both physically and mentally, if we follow His counsel contained in the Word of Wisdom. He has made it simple and non-cumbersome to follow, so that all may reap the benefits of His wisdom and knowledge. You don't have to be a genius to follow His code of health; you only need knowledge and the desire to do so.

We live in a time where profit and wealth is considered over health and wellness; a time where many "conspiring men" produce and sell products that adversely affect health, despite having full knowledge that these products are unhealthy. Selfish and greedy men pad their wallets to the detriment of those who consume their products. Misleading and fraudulent advertisements are created by cunning men in order to create desirability for their products. The consequence of this is poor health. An example of this is a study published in the Annals of Internal Medicine indicating the need for long-term use of smoking cessation products, despite the fact these same products are known to have side effects such as suicidal thoughts, seizures, and loss of consciousness. The four experts that conducted the research were funded by the manufacturers of smoking cessation products that had billions of dollars to gain by getting such a report published. This appears to be nothing more than telling the pharmaceutical companies what they want to hear, in order to generate billions of more dollars in profits. Even Harvard Medical School has recently indicated that they feel the influence of pharmaceutical companies is too prevalent in their schools, because of the millions of dollars these companies pour into this educational institution.

Conspiring men are not new to earth. Benefiting from conspiracy existed among our earliest ancestors. As noted in the bible, Cain killed his brother Abel for gain. The father of all lies used man's appetite for greed against Cain, and Cain paid dearly for it. Satan continues his desire and purpose of creating misery for man today. He uses the same desire for gain and "conspiring men" as his pawns in his wicked game to inflict disease, sickness, pain, misery, and death upon man. Ultimately, Satan's goal is to separate man from God. His methods are very subtle and often difficult to detect.

The cigarette industry is an appropriate example of "conspiring men". They concealed and obscured evidence that cigarettes were unhealthy and had been implicated in many chronic illnesses. Phillip Morris, the largest cigarette manufacture in the world, knew at least by the 1980s that secondhand smoke was extremely toxic, but hid this truth for decades[12]. They covered up this information because they did not want their product to be adversely affected. There was no thought for human health, only thought for protection of profits. They did not want to lose their gain, despite the destruction it was proliferating among men. Smoking is not nearly as glamorous when you see someone breathing through a tube in his or her neck as a result of the adverse effects of smoking. The only reason for the existence of a product such as cigarettes is to provide profit to government agencies through taxes, and the cigarette manufacturers. Why else would a product linked to cancer, heart disease, stroke, emphysema, and premature death be allowed to continue on the market? The government has pulled other products for lesser offenses than this, but it continues to turn a blind eye toward the cigarette industry.

Other harmful substances have been portrayed as socially acceptable by various means. Television and movie shows are full of instances where drugs and alcohol are portrayed as customary. People try to justify the use of drugs for medicinal purposes, when better alternatives are clearly available. Advertising and marketing campaigns bombard us with promotions to represent alcohol, smoking, and other harmful products as normal and even cool. It is imperative that we stand firm in avoiding harmful substances and not yield to these addicting and health deteriorating products. If we stand firm, we will be able to avoid the trap of being addicted to harmful products. Some products are so powerful that trying them once can create a biological craving for the product. This creates a physical addiction that is almost impossible for some to overcome. The addicted person becomes hopeless and forlorn, with little hope of conquering such a gripping addiction.

How often have we seen businesses collapse because of the unsavory actions of managers, executives, and owners? The financial crisis of 2008 was largely due to executives manipulating their companies' accounting books so that they could receive their bonuses. In an effort to keep up with the Jones's, people cheat, embezzle, lie, and steal. Moral decency, honesty, and integrity have been replaced by greed, power, and wealth. Man's desire for profit that existed in the time of Adam continues wholeheartedly today. The term 'conspiring men' is applicable to more than just the manufacturers of addictive drugs and products. This term could easily be applied to any person who willingly sells a harmful product for gain.

The fast food industry is a good example of conspiring men, but is not often thought of in that way. The fast food companies continue to advertise and market their products despite established adverse health effects. They sell products that are full of calories, fat, sugar, and salt, which contribute to the poor health of Americans. In this day and age of instant information, do they really expect us to believe that they don't know the food they sell contributes to negative health consequences? Absolutely not. They know about the detrimental effects of the food they sell, but choose to ignore them for the sake of profits.

With circumstances such as these, is it any wonder that God sent the Word of Wisdom by greeting and not by commandment? If He had sent it by commandment at the time of the revelation, countless numbers of people would have come under immediate condemnation because of their addictions. Instead, the Lord provided a period of time for His saints to familiarize themselves with the revelation and to relinquish problematic addictions. He, in His usual loving and kind way, sent the Word of Wisdom to give us counsel, guidance, and direction, while still giving us time to overcome addictions to unhealthful products and habits. After sufficient time had passed, church president Brigham Young announced that the revelation was a command of the Lord[13] and that members of the church are now expected to live by its precepts.

We are told that our body is a temple (1 Corinthians 3:16). Should we not then treat our body as we would treat the temple of God? How many of us would bring toxic and poisonous substances into the temple with the full knowledge that they would harm the temple? We need to take care of our bodies and respect the creation of our Maker by listening to and obeying His counsel. Many of us take better care of our vehicles than we do of our bodies. If a vehicle manufacturer recommends oil changes at regular intervals (which all of them do), we take our vehicle to be serviced at regular intervals. We rely upon the owner's manual to tell us how to best take care of our vehicles, yet we disregard the manual the Lord has provided for our bodies. What a tragedy it is that we have our owner's manual in front of us, yet choose to leave it on the shelf, ignoring the instructions contained therein. If this same practice were applied to our vehicles, they would quickly deteriorate and fail. This is the exact path that those who choose to ignore the Word of Wisdom are following – one in which their bodies will deteriorate and break down. Our bodies require proper care and nourishment to function optimally.

Chapter 2

Doctrine & Covenants 89:5-7 & 9

"That inasmuch as any man drinketh wine or strong drink among you, behold it is not good, neither meet in the sight of your Father, only in assembling yourselves together to offer up your sacraments before him.

And, behold, this should be wine, yea, pure wine of the grape of the vine, of your own make.

And again strong drinks are not for the belly, but for the washing of your bodies.

And again, hot drinks are not for the body or the belly."

Families are torn apart and lives are lost from the abuse of alcohol. Alcohol is a drug and central nervous system depressant. Alcohol is a poison, harmful to the organs of the body. It suppresses inhibitions and moral sense and therefore the ability to appropriately control one's self. Character is weakened and immoral acts are more likely when under its influence. Even small amounts of alcohol can change behavior, generally making the consumer more careless and irresponsible under its influence. Many people do things under the influence of alcohol that they would not normally do. Alcohol gives us a false sense of well-being while decreasing motor skills, decreasing muscle control, reducing coordination, impairing judgment, and retarding ability to reason. This is why people under the influence of alcohol drive so erratically and why their speech is slurred.

Unfortunately, the actions of those who choose to drive while impaired with alcohol or other substances greatly affect the lives of others on a daily basis. Not only do they ruin their health and lives, but they also do the same to others. Alcohol consumption is the third leading preventable cause of death in the United States[14]. Every day, more than 207 deaths are attributed to this destructive drug[15]. Alcohol can often lead to behavioral changes such as anger and violence – just ask the children or spouse of an angry drunk. The home of a drunk is no place for children. Often children in this situation will seek solace at the house of a friend to avoid the negative interaction with their father or mother. The Lord knows the negative consequences of drinking alcohol and strong drinks and therefore warns us not to partake of them.

Alcohol is a very addictive drug and a voracious appetite may be acquired with its continual use. Many people are slaves to this addiction and both they and their families suffer because of it. There are numerous helpful programs to overcome this addiction, including a program instituted by the Church of Jesus Christ of Latter Day Saints. However, it is so much better to avoid alcohol completely, thus avoiding the addiction altogether.

The costs of alcohol addiction are enormous, financially and physically, to both individuals and families. Some are so addicted to alcohol they seek a temporary buzz from the content of odd sources such as vanilla extracts, cough syrup, and even rubbing alcohol. Commonly, this method is used by those not of legal age, such as teenagers. This destructive routine only leads a person down a more destructive path as they try to satisfy their addiction.

There are many negative effects of alcohol consumption on your health. Because alcohol is a diuretic, it causes rapid water loss. If you are drinking alcohol for hydration, think again. Alcohol leaches water from your system and does not provide it. Alcohol depletes vitamins and minerals from your body, particularly magnesium, folic acid, vitamin B12, thiamine, pyridoxine (vitamin B6), vitamin A, and zinc. All of these vitamins and minerals play critical roles in the processes and function of your body. Excessive alcohol consumption can lead to deficiencies in these key nutrients and to the diseases related to their deficiency. Excessive alcohol consumption can lead to liver cirrhosis, various cancers, and unintentional injuries. Alcohol irritates the intestines and the liver, the primary organ of detoxification. The liver attempts to detoxify alcohol from the body, but when it gets overwhelmed, liver cells may be destroyed or damaged, leading to fat deposits in the liver, liver inflammation, or permanent scarring (cirrhosis). If the liver is damaged, body toxicity can result because the liver is unable to rid the body of the toxins.

Much information has been published about the health benefits of moderate wine consumption, especially red wine. There is some truth to these assertions. However, what the studies, and especially the wine industry, fail to inform you is that you can receive the same benefits from consuming grape juice. These wine studies are contradictory in nature, with one claiming health benefits such as reduced risk of heart disease[16], while another claims wine doubles the risk of breast cancer[17]. Which should you believe? The Lord has provided the definitive answer. Wine and alcohol should not be consumed.

The benefits that are derived from wine consumption are a result of the phytochemicals, antioxidants, and flavonoids contained in grapes, particularly the skin of grapes. In fact, the concentration of the flavonoid resveratrol is much higher in a serving of grapes (including the grape skins) than it is in wine itself. Red wine contains from 1.5 to 3.0 milligrams of resveratrol per liter, while fresh grape skins contain 5 to 10 milligrams per serving[18].

To better understand what antioxidants do in the body, we must have a discussion about free radicals. Free radicals are molecules produced during the normal energy-producing processes within our cells. Cells normally contain biochemicals that have paired electrons. When these biochemicals are missing an electron, they become free radicals, and thus go on a rampage to capture an electron from other cell components, such as DNA, thus damaging it. When a cell's DNA is damaged, it is able to mutate, grow, and reproduce abnormally and rapidly. The end result is illness or disease. Free radicals may originate from metabolism, inflammation, stress, and exposure to toxic chemicals. In fact, your body's immune system uses free radicals in the process of destroying foreign bodies such as viruses and bacteria. The same process that damages healthy cells also damages bacteria and viruses.

Antioxidants prevent damage to cells within your body. Oxygen is critical to life, but plays a damaging role as well. If you have ever seen the rusting (oxidation) that takes place when metal is left exposed to the elements, imagine that process now taking place inside your body. Not a pretty sight to imagine, is it? Another example of oxidation is when apple or banana slices turn brown when exposed to oxygen. If oxidation is left unchecked, it eventually damages cells to the point they no longer function correctly. This malfunction can then lead to cancer, heart disease, diabetes, and many other conditions. Antioxidants work in a chemical process and exchange electrons to neutralize this oxidation process, but they only work when there is adequate supply and continual renewal of the antioxidants. In an effort to combat the oxidation process, antioxidants are oxidized themselves, and they require replenishment by another antioxidant to continue the battle. The body's need for antioxidants is dependent on its current condition. For example, someone with arthritis or another chronic illness will have greater requirements for antioxidants than someone who does not have those ailments.

Flavonoids are complex chemicals contained within plants, especially in fruits, vegetables, and whole grains. They act as powerful antioxidants within the body, assisting in the battle against free radicals. Some scientists and doctors believe that flavonoids may hold the key to controlling cancer, both as a preventative and as a treatment[19]. Grapes contain the flavonoid resveratrol which is an outstanding antioxidant and has the ability to lower LDL (bad cholesterol), and reduce the risk of heart disease. Other important phytochemicals found in grapes that work in the battle against free radicals are proanthocyanidins, saponins, and anthocyanins.

Alcohol has been implicated as a contributing factor in heart disease, high blood pressure, heart failure, and stroke. Drinking too much of it can raise triglyceride (fats in the blood) levels[20]. High triglyceride levels are associated with greater risk of heart disease. Alcohol is not meant for internal consumption, rather for external use only. It is best to keep alcohol to its intended use as an antiseptic "to wash our bodies". In this function, it inhibits growth of many microorganisms, including viruses, bacteria, and fungi.

We have been told that the term "strong drinks" also includes coffee and tea. Joseph Smith, as quoted by Joel H. Johnson, stated "[Tea and coffee] are what the Lord meant when he said 'hot drinks'"[21]. This is also a logical assumption, because the common "hot drinks" of Joseph Smith's time were coffee and tea. Brigham Young spoke of this when he said "I have heard it argued that tea and coffee are not mentioned [in the Word of Wisdom]; that is very true; but what were the people in the habit of taking as hot drinks when the revelation was given? Tea and coffee. We were not in the habit of drinking water very hot, but tea and coffee-the beverages in common use"[22]. In addition, Victor Ludlow asserts "The Word of Wisdom counsels against drinking 'hot drinks', which have been identified by early church leaders as coffee and tea. 'Tea' refers to the standard tea derived from the tea plant, sometimes called black or green tea. The Word of Wisdom has not been interpreted as proscribing herbal teas, stating that 'all wholesome herbs God hath ordained for the constitution, nature, and use of man (D&C 89:10)".[23]

Because statements have been made that tea is against the Word of Wisdom, we have made tea a negative word among Latter-Day Saints. We do not differentiate between beneficial herbal teas and standard teas, simply stating that all tea is against the word of wisdom. Why, if God has stated that herbs are beneficial for man, would we assume that they are not beneficial when consumed in tea form? This goes against all logic and reason. Technically any plant having leaves that are boiled in water to create a beverage could be considered a tea. Does this mean if you boil carrot leaves and drink the water you are breaking the Word of Wisdom?

While all coffee (yes even decaffeinated) and some teas contain the drug caffeine, there are many other substances to be concerned about in these common beverages; namely the xanthine alkaloids theophylline and theobromine, the tannins they contain, fluoride, chlorogenic acid, and oxalate.

Although the Word of Wisdom does not specifically forbid caffeine, Bishop H. Burke Peterson had the following to say about it. "We should notice the word wholesome and always consider the things that we take into our body as to whether they are wholesome or not. The scripture continues 'All these to be used with prudence and thanksgiving' (D&C 89:11)....We know that cola drinks contain the drug caffeine. We know that caffeine is not wholesome nor prudent for the use of our bodies. It is only sound judgment to conclude that cola drinks and others that contain caffeine or other harmful ingredients should not be used"[24]. Drinks that contain harmful and habit-forming drugs should therefore be avoided. It is important for everyone to prayerfully consider what this indicates to them, as the Lord will not command in all things. He leaves us room to make our own decisions and choices, and will not force anyone to live healthily.

Caffeine is the most abused behavior-modifying drug in the world. In excessive amounts, caffeine is addictive, causes jumpiness and heart palpitations, reduces mental function, can restrict liver function, reduces fertility in women, causes headaches in some people, leaches B vitamins from the body, and depletes essential minerals (especially calcium) from the body[25]. When caffeine first enters the bloodstream, it is very stimulating, but after its immediate effects wear off, it actually depresses the system. This up and then down effect deceives the user into believing that they feel better when under the influence of caffeine. It provides a false sense of more energy and liveliness. Because caffeine is a stimulant, it may cause insomnia as well as hyperactivity. The list of negative effects of caffeine continues, with osteoporosis, diarrhea, increased blood pressure, increased cholesterol and triglyceride levels, fibrocystic breast disease, birth defects and miscarriages, kidney stones, increased incidence of some cancers, prostate enlargement, adrenal exhaustion, increased heartburn, and anxiety.[26] Why anyone would want to consume large quantities of a drink that contains such a destructive drug each day is unfathomable.

Is it any wonder that Americans are plagued with health problems when we drink caffeinated soda, coffee, and teas as water substitutes? I know many people who feel they could not make it through the day without indulging in these unhealthy beverages. They have to make trip after trip to the pop or coffee machine to maintain the feeling of energy that they lose when not consuming caffeinated beverages. Their bodies have become used to having these stimulants and in many ways now require them. The brain receives craving signals from the body for these substances because of their addictive nature. It is wise to slowly wean yourself from these addictive substances, because quitting abruptly can cause severe withdrawal symptoms. In addition, the sugary syrup contained in soda drinks creates more desire to consume them freely, making them in some ways worse than coffee and tea that are consumed slowly because of their bitter flavor.

Recently, energy drinks have become very popular. Unfortunately, these drinks provide energy by injecting significant quantities of caffeine into the bloodstream. These drinks are targeted to teens, despite a warning label on some of them that indicates they should not be consumed by anyone under age eighteen. One energy drink even boasts of three hundred milligrams of caffeine in one 8.4 ounce serving. Sadly, caffeinism, or an overdose of caffeine, can occur with as little as two hundred and fifty milligrams. The FDA limits the amount of caffeine contained in food products to seventy-one milligrams per twelve ounces. However, energy drinks are labeled as dietary supplements and so don't fall under these restrictions. Energy drink manufacturers go unchecked, loading their products with as much of this addictive substance as possible, thus creating the desire to consume more and more of the product. Five to six hundred milligrams of caffeine can cause anxiety, muscle tremors, and abnormal heart rhythms. Recently many people have succumbed to the caffeine content of these energy drinks and have been hospitalized. Even athletes in superb shape are not immune to an overdose of caffeine. Energy drinks have even been implicated as a contributing factor in a few deaths.

Black and green teas originate from the same tea (*Camellia sinensis*) plant. They differ in the manner in which they are processed. Black tea is processed further than green tea through fermentation. Fermentation is the oxidation of the plant polyphenols in the tea leaf. Green tea has received rave press regarding its antioxidant properties, which indeed it has. It is also touted as a weight loss miracle. Green tea contains powerful antioxidants and is used medicinally for many purposes. However, looking only at green tea's antioxidant properties dismisses the hundreds of other biochemical compounds it contains, and their possible health benefits and risks. The tea plant contains the xanthine alkaloids caffeine, theobromine, and theophylline, all of which are central nervous system stimulants and diuretics. The tea plant also contains significant amounts of fluoride, tannin, and some oxalate. Dr. Clifford Stratton states "The xanthines stimulate the brain and spinal cord, increase heart action, constrict blood vessels feeding the brain (that's why extra-strength aspirin compounds help a headache so dramatically), relieve respiratory distress by relaxing certain muscles, strengthen the contractions of arm and leg muscles, increase the production of urine, increase the amount of acid secreted into the stomach, and generally increase body metabolism"[27]. Too many xanthines in the system may cause diarrhea, dizziness, trembling, frequent urination, and insomnia.

There are some people who believe it is ok to drink iced tea because it is not a "hot drink". However, they are incorrect in this thinking, because iced tea is often derived from the *Camellia sinensis* plant and it carries the same health risks. Just because it is not hot does not mean it is not prohibited by the Word of Wisdom. All drinks that are injurious or addictive should be avoided. Moreover, even drinks that are too hot can damage the mouth, tongue, and esophagus, and they should be consumed with great caution.

Excessive tea consumption stimulates overproduction of gastric acid and may lead to indigestion. In addition, too much tea may lead to kidney stones because of its oxalate content. The stimulants in the tea plant may also over-stimulate the kidneys, causing permanent damage. It appears that theobromine is more irritating to the kidneys than is caffeine. Excessive tea consumption has been linked with aggravating premenstrual symptoms[28] and may lead to incontinence, and frequent or urgent impulses to urinate[29].

Theobromine is suspected of being toxic to the endocrine system (the body system comprised of organs and glands that secrete hormones to control normal physiological processes), toxic to the liver and gastrointestinal tract, a neurotoxin (substances that cause adverse affects on the central nervous system), and has been implicated as a contributing factor in adverse effects to the reproductive system.[30] Because of its diuretic nature, it increases the body's requirement for fluid.

Theophylline's negative effects are similar to those of caffeine, only it is considered slightly more toxic. It stimulates the heart and respiratory system. Because it is a bronchodilator, it is sometimes used medicinally in the treatment of asthma. Theophylline may make you irritable, nauseous, or give you a headache. When combined, theobromine, caffeine, and theophylline strengthen their diuretic and stimulant properties. The power and strength of this combination can result in more frequent and serious adverse side effects.

The chlorogenic acid content in coffee and black tea increases plasma homocysteine levels, a predictor of cardiovascular disease[31]. This indicates that increased consumption of coffee and black tea increases the risk of heart disease. Americans could realize a significant reduction in the risk of heart disease by eliminating these two harmful drinks that are so frequently consumed.

Some people switch from coffee to tea, believing it to be a healthier beverage. Unfortunately, they are not achieving their goal of a healthier beverage to consume. The adverse effects of tea from the *Camellia sinensis* plant are similar to those of coffee. The *Camellia sinensis* plant contains high amounts of naturally occurring fluoride, derived from air and soil pollution. The Environmental Protection Agency has set the drinking standard for fluoride at four milligrams per liter, and a secondary standard of two milligrams per liter to protect against dental fluorosis[32]. Dental fluorosis is a condition caused by excessive intake of fluoride, resulting in mottling of the teeth. One liter of green or black tea contains anywhere from 1.0mg to 1.9mg of fluoride alone. The average green tea bottle contains approximately one half liter, and one eight-ounce cup of black tea is equivalent to almost one-quarter liter. These figures indicate that many people are drinking enough tea to consume an unhealthy amount of fluoride every day. This is also assuming that the water they use to make the tea is not fluoridated. If the water is fluoridated, the level of fluoride increases dramatically, as does the toxicity of the tea. Astonishingly, fluoride is more poisonous than lead. In excessive amounts it has been linked to cancer, Alzheimer's, poor brain development in children, decreased thyroid activity, increased risk of bone fractures, atherosclerosis, dental fluorosis, and nervous system problems[33].

Product	Caffeine (mg)
Coffee (6 oz. cup)	
Drip	175
Percolated	132
Instant regular	62
Decaffeinated	2
Tea	
Black	47
Green	30-50
White	15
Soft Drinks (12 oz. can)	
Mountain Dew	54
Dr. Pepper	47
Pepsi	38
Diet Coke	47
Energy Drinks	
Full Throttle (16 oz.)	144
Monster (16 oz.)	160
Candy Bars	
Hershey Bar (1.55 oz)	9

Resource: USDA National Nutrient Database for Standard Reference, 2007.

Tannins are defensive chemicals found in plants used as protection from consumption by predators. The same substance that gives tea its bitter flavor wards off animals who may otherwise consume it. Coffee contains smaller quantities of tannic acid than tea. The tannin content in tea increases according to the age of the leaf. The older the leaf, the more tannin it contains. About seven to fourteen percent of tea leaf composition is tannins. Research has shown a correlation between tannin and cancer of the esophagus[34]. Tannic acid can also cause indigestion and stomach ulcers. I find it ironic that we freely consume a chemical meant to ward off animals and insects.

Millions of people start their day with a cup of coffee. They continue drinking this beverage throughout the day, cup after cup. The caffeine content in coffee makes it a significant contributor to caffeine abuse. This is such a common beverage and practice that many see the LDS churches restriction of coffee as very odd. Coffee is such a strong drink that it often creates chemical dependence. Physical symptoms of withdrawal, including headache, difficulty concentrating, and fatigue, are common when the usual dose of coffee is reduced. The same three xanthine alkaloids (theobromine, theophylline, and caffeine) are contained in coffee, so the same effects are expected. One big difference is that coffee contains significantly more caffeine than does tea; depending on the coffee, almost four times more than black tea, and more than five times the amount in green tea. (See table) According to Dr. Kaslow, the following are health issues associated with coffee and caffeine: exhausted adrenal glands (the stimulating effect of caffeine causes the adrenals to secrete the hormone adrenaline, overuse of which exhausts them); severe blood sugar swings; acid imbalance (coffee stimulates the secretion of acid in the stomach, optimal health calls for an alkaline pH balance to the body); and essential mineral depletion (coffee causes the excretion of some minerals in the urine and inhibits the absorption of others)[35]. One of the minerals that coffee reduces the absorption of is non-heme iron (iron from plant sources), which increases the risk of anemia. The regular consumption of coffee may lead to cardiac sensitivity, abnormal heartbeats, anxiety, irritability, intestinal irritation, and insomnia[36].

Some choose to eliminate caffeine from their coffee and drink decaffeinated coffee. However, the chemicals used to decaffeinate coffee create additional health concerns, particularly the large amounts of hydrogen peroxide it contains. Frankly, there just isn't a healthful type of coffee to drink.

When it comes to healthy beverages, water reigns supreme. Nothing quenches thirst as well as water. Purified drinking water is even better because it eliminates many of the heavy metals, microorganisms, and chemicals that are unfortunately contained in drinking water. A good rule of thumb is to drink six to eight, eight ounce glasses of water per day. Don't wait until you're thirsty to drink water. When your body has insufficient water, it sends this thirst signal so that you will drink the water it needs. This can be difficult in our busy and distracting lives, but is critical to our health. I find it easy to accomplish this amount of water consumption by keeping a bottle of water at my desk to drink from throughout the day. Water is fundamental to life as the primary component of all bodily fluids, including blood, lymph, tears, urine, sweat, and digestive juices. Water is essential to remove waste products of metabolism. In addition, water is involved in almost every bodily function, including most chemical reactions and the many life processes that take place in water. Our cells rely upon sufficient water to function properly.

Other healthy beverages are fruit and vegetable juices. However, be careful of commercial juices, which are full of added sugar. Juicing your own fresh fruit and vegetables is by far the healthiest and best method. This allows you to know exactly what is in your juice and to control how much sugar is added, if any. Fruits are naturally high in sugar and will taste sweet without the addition of refined sugar. Add apples or other sweet fruits to your vegetables to make them sweeter and more palatable. Juicing releases numerous health-promoting phytochemicals, including flavonoids beneficial for your health. When you make your own juice, you preserve good quantities of vitamins and some minerals. If you don't want to invest in a juicer or don't think that you have the time, look for unsweetened juice at a health food store.

Chapter 3

Doctrine and Covenants 89:8

"And again, tobacco is not for the body, neither for the belly, and is not good for man, but as an herb for bruises and all sick cattle, to be used with judgment and skill."

Ironically, the government works vigorously to protect us from air pollution while turning a blind eye to toxic and dangerous tobacco products. This fact is utterly astonishing and another indication of the evil designs of conspiring men. Tobacco smoke contains more than four thousand chemicals[37], of which eighty-one, so far, have been identified as cancer causing[38]. Why anyone in their right mind would submit their body to this toxic assault is beyond reason. Each puff wreaks havoc within the body as the body tries to detoxify an overabundance of unhealthy and toxic chemicals.

Most historians credit the Native Americans for instituting the use of tobacco for smoking. Christopher Columbus observed the Indians in this practice when he discovered the Americas. In the mid 1900s, smoking was portrayed as being glamorous by movie stars, athletes, and political figures who were constantly seen smoking. All the while, the cigarette companies were producing massive quantities of a toxic product and earning significant profits at the expense of the smoker's health. Considerable amounts of money were spent advertising cigarettes as sophisticated and prestigious, even healthful (for their appetite suppressing effect), and unfortunately, some of this advertising appeared to be geared toward teenagers and children. Many can remember the cartoon character Joe Camel that was used to market cigarettes. This was an obvious ploy to interest the young in this deplorable habit. These marketing programs, as well as the suppression of the scientific research implicating cigarettes to disease, were very successful. It didn't take long for tobacco companies to secure a sizeable, addicted population to which they could sell their product.

Cigarette smoking is the most preventable cause of premature death and is a major single cause of cancer mortality in the United States. In fact, cigarette smoking accounts for at least thirty percent of all cancer deaths, and eighty-seven percent of lung cancer deaths[39]. The United States Department of Health and Human Services found that smoking is accountable for ninety percent of lung cancers in men, and seventy-nine percent in women[40]. It is a major cause of lung, larynx (voice box), oral cavity, pharynx (throat), esophagus, and bladder cancers, and contributes to stomach, cervix, kidney, and pancreas cancers, as well as some leukemias. The smoker's risk of developing these cancers increases with the number of cigarettes smoked each day, the age that smoking was commenced, and the duration of the smoker's lifetime spent smoking. Think of the reduction in lung cancer deaths attributed to smoking if smokers would heed these warnings and give up the habit. Significant medical and scientific research is available that publicizes the health benefits of smoking cessation. Amazingly, one person dies almost every minute from illnesses related to cigarette smoking in the United States. This accounts for about one in five deaths in the country[41].

Smoking harms almost every organ of the body, causes or contributes to a great many diseases, and reduces quality of life. Smoking contributes to heart disease, bronchitis, emphysema, stroke, aneurysms, high cholesterol, pneumonia, influenza, the common cold, chronic bowel disease, peptic ulcers, tooth decay, gum disease, osteoporosis, thyroid disease, cataracts, and bronchitis[42]. It is damaging to reproductive health, especially in women. Smoking is linked with reduced fertility, increased risk of miscarriage, premature births, low birth-weight infants, stillbirth, and infant death. Smoking is a detriment to physical fitness and endurance, because it reduces the ability of the blood to carry oxygen. The Center for Disease Control estimates that male chronic smokers lose an average of 13.2 years of life expectancy, while female chronic smokers lose 14.5[43]. Taking into account current average life expectancy, this equals approximately fifteen percent of a smoker's life.

Instead of dying as a direct result of smoking, many people suffer through life with a debilitating chronic illness, which significantly reduces their quality of life. They may have to carry an oxygen tank everywhere they go to provide sufficient oxygen to the body. They may suffer reduced quality of life from coronary heart disease or stroke. A smoker's quality of life is very often reduced during the "golden years", if not earlier.

Ironically, people smoke despite the immediate detrimental effects that are felt when smoking for the first time. A person's first use of tobacco generally causes illness. The body attempts to rid itself of nicotine through expulsion, including coughing and vomiting. As the person smokes more cigarettes, and as nicotine is continually introduced to the body, a tolerance is built up. Once body tolerance sets in, addiction is likely.

The three chemicals contained in cigarettes that are most worrisome appear to be nicotine, tar, and carbon monoxide. We increasingly place carbon monoxide detectors in our home to avoid exposure to this toxic killer, yet we allow people to inhale it in cigarettes every day. How many of us would line up to place our mouth over our car's exhaust pipe? Yet we introduce the same toxic chemical into our bodies through smoking cigarettes. Carbon monoxide is a silent killer that we should strive to avoid in any form.

Many of the chemicals that are used in various industries are found in cigarettes. We wear protective equipment to avoid exposure to these chemicals, but they are readily accessible in cigarettes. It is ironic that government agencies would fine industries for allowing employees to come in unprotected contact with the same chemicals found in cigarettes, yet allows smokers to inhale them on a daily basis. One would think that cigarettes would be banned outright, or at least controlled more ardently, given the plethora of harmful chemicals contained in them. I believe an employer would find it hard to convince the Occupational Safety Hazard Association that their employees would be safe coming in contact with the same plethora of chemicals during the workday. Rather than bore you with scientific data about all four-thousand chemicals in cigarettes, I will give a brief overview of some of the most harmful chemicals they contain.

Tar, a black sticky product used to cover road surfaces, clogs the lungs and causes lung cancer. Some of the carcinogenic (cancer causing) chemicals contained in tar are:

- Benzopyrene – When exposed to this chemical in the short term, it has been shown to potentially cause red blood cell damage, leading to anemia, and to suppress the immune system. Long-term exposure has the potential to cause reproductive and developmental damage, and cancer[44].

- B-naphthylamine – used in the manufacture of dyes and rubber, this product causes kidney, liver, and brain damage.
- Cadmium – is an extremely poisonous metal commonly found in manufacturing facilities where car batteries are made, or ore is smelted or processed. Even trace amounts of this metal can produce unhealthy effects. Acute inhalation may result in long lasting impairment of lung function, while chronic exposure can result in kidney, lung, liver, bone, immune system, blood, and nervous system damage[45].
- Tobacco-Specific N-Nitrosamine – In animal studies, nitrosamines are considered one of the most powerful carcinogens. While more research needs to be conducted regarding their full effects on humans, I believe it is safe to say that nitrosamines are unhealthful for humans as well. They have been linked to oral, lung, liver, pancreatic, and esophageal cancer[46].

Nicotine, a poisonous alkaloid, is the addictive drug contained within cigarettes. Nicotine travels through the bloodstream and to the brain in a matter of seconds. This powerful drug is a stimulant that raises heart rate and blood pressure and increases the stickiness of blood vessels, which in turn increases the risk of heart attack and stroke. Nicotine creates a terrible physical and psychological addiction. Many people attempt to quit smoking each year, but fewer than five percent succeed[47]. The physical and emotional addictions of this drug are extremely difficult to overcome. Despite knowing the injurious effects of this habit, smokers have great difficulty quitting. Their addiction becomes more powerful than their desire to live a healthful life and reduce risk of disease. Smokers certainly have not been helped by cigarette manufacturers. According to one report, these "conspiring men" knowingly and deliberately have increased the nicotine levels in cigarettes[48]. Of course, the tobacco industry vehemently denies this allegation, but they also denied that their products were addictive and unhealthy, until they were forced to admit they are detrimental to health.

You may think that carbon monoxide only comes from car exhaust, but you would be wrong in this assumption. This deadly poison, found in cigarette smoke, robs the muscles, brain, and body tissue of oxygen, causing your heart to work harder. This overworking of the heart can cause heart attack and stroke, and over time, causes swelling of the airways, which lets less air into the lungs. Carbon monoxide is an odorless and colorless gas – a silent but very deadly killer. At lower levels of exposure, carbon monoxide causes headache, dizziness, nausea, fatigue, and disorientation[49]. Carbon monoxide inhibits oxygen intake by creating carboxyhemoglobin in the blood. As your body's tissues starve of oxygen, detrimental effects occur. At moderate concentrations, it may cause angina (heart pain), impaired vision, and reduced brain function. Very high concentrations can be fatal[50].

How many of us would line up to ingest chemicals used as household cleaning products and fertilizers? Yet this is exactly what smokers do through the inhalation of ammonia contained in cigarettes. Unfortunately, the cigarette companies use ammonia to boost the impact of nicotine in cigarettes. This process of adding ammonia to cigarettes is similar to the process of using chemicals to heighten the effects of cocaine, called "free-basing". Ammonia helps convert nicotine from its acid to base form, allowing it to more fully and quickly diffuse through the body. The cigarette companies know that nicotine is the addictive chemical in cigarettes and want to make it more addictive through this process. Again, this is done without regard to health consequences, simply to increase the saleability of the product and thus profits. The more addicted smokers that can be created, the more profit that is produced. Ammonia is an eye, nose, skin, and throat irritant and has the following potential health effects: asthma, acute lung damage, and blindness[51].

Arsenic is a naturally occurring compound found throughout the environment. It is used in ammunition manufacturing to make bullets harder and rounder. It is used in tanning and taxidermy as a preservative, and as a wood surface preservative and treatment. Much concern has been expressed over the use of arsenic in the treatment of wood used in playground equipment. Industries that use this compound must take great care to avoid exposure and the adverse health effects associated with it. It has been shown to cause diarrhea, nausea, abdominal pain, central and peripheral nervous system disorders, skin and mucous membrane irritation, anemia, peripheral neuropathy, skin lesions, kidney and liver damage, and lung, liver, and bladder cancer[52].

Benzene is a highly flammable, colorless liquid found in coal and oil burning emissions, gasoline at service stations, and car exhaust. It has a very high melting point, and a sweet odor. It has been used as a gasoline additive, pesticide, detergent, dye, lubricant, degreaser, and in explosives. In fact, this toxic chemical was also used to decaffeinate coffee at one point. Benzene may cause drowsiness, dizziness, headaches, eye, skin, and respiratory irritation, unconsciousness, reduction in the number of red blood cells, harm to the female reproductive system, and an increased incidence of leukemia (cancer of the tissues that form white blood cells)[53].

Cadmium is a soft transitional metal largely used in batteries and pigments and as a plastic stabilizer. Cadmium exposure may cause a number of harmful health effects in humans. These include irritation and damage to the lungs, kidney damage, the formation of kidney stones, and death[54]. In animal studies, cadmium has been shown to cause high blood pressure, iron-poor blood, liver disease, nerve and brain damage[55].

Chloroform was originally used as an anesthetic during surgery in the mid 1800s. Soon after its use, sudden deaths during anesthesia were reported. Because of these reports, and with the advent of safer anesthetics, chloroform fell out of favor. Chloroform is also used in laundry starch, paint-related products, automotive chemicals, pesticides, and specialty cleaning and sanitation products. The predominant use today is for the production of air conditioning refrigerant, but recent environmental legislation will reduce and eliminate this use, as refrigerants become more environmentally friendly. Unfortunately, chloroform can be released into the air as a result of its formation in chlorinated drinking water and swimming pools. Its major health effect is central nervous system depression, but it also may cause liver problems (including hepatitis, tumors, and jaundice), and kidney tumors[56].

Formaldehyde, the same chemical that morticians use to embalm deceased individuals, is also found in cigarettes. It is a colorless gas with a very pungent odor. The various forms of formaldehyde are used as a preservative and disinfectant, in pressed wood products (its highest concentration level), foam insulation, carpets, clothing, and some appliances. It can cause watery, burning eyes and a burning sensation in the throat. In addition, it can cause nausea, seizures, coma, liver and kidney damage, headache, central nervous system damage, and dermatitis[57]. Animal studies have demonstrated effects on the lungs, spleen, liver, and thyroid and increased incidence of lung, nasal cavity, and liver tumors[58].

Lead remains one of the greatest environmental health hazards in the United States. It is most dangerous to children because of the likelihood that they will touch a lead object and then put their hands in their mouths. In addition, children seem to absorb lead more readily than do adults, and their developing brain and nervous system are more susceptible to its damaging effects. The government banned the use of leaded gasoline to protect us from exposure, but continues to allow cigarettes that contain lead to be sold. Regrettably, many homes built prior to 1978 have lead-based paint that is harmful to children. Lead based paint was banned by the federal government in 1978. Recently, toys manufactured in China have been exposed for the use of lead-based paint. That a manufacturer would allow toys that will without a doubt end up in children's mouths to be coated with a deadly toxin is unconscionable – but, then again, the cigarette industry does the same thing; by knowingly supplying a lead-containing product that ultimately ends up in the mouths of adults. Exposure to lead may also come from contaminated soil, which gets its lead content from lead-based paint or past use of leaded gasoline. Drinking water is another source of lead, especially if your home has plumbing with lead pipes or soldering.

Lead is primarily used in the manufacture of lead-acid storage batteries, but it is also used in alloys, ammunition, foil, as cable coverings, in the lining of laboratory sinks, and in the protective shielding against x-ray and radiation. It may cause brain and nervous system damage, behavior and learning disabilities, hyperactivity, impeded growth, hearing problems, headaches, reproductive problems (both men and women), high blood pressure, nerve disorders, memory and concentration problems, and muscle and joint pain[59].

Vinyl chloride is primarily used in the production of PVC (polyvinyl chloride) plastic and vinyl products. It was once used as an aerosol spray propellant in products like hair spray, and briefly as an inhalational anesthetic; although this practice was discontinued when its toxicity was discovered. Exposure to vinyl chloride can result in central nervous system problems such as dizziness, drowsiness, and headaches; and other health effects like liver damage and cancer[60].

Sadly, those who choose to smoke don't just affect themselves, but also anyone else who is exposed to the byproduct of their smoking, secondhand smoke; also known as environmental tobacco smoke (ETS). Smokers are so addicted to their habit that they often expose someone they love and care about to ETS. I am dismayed when I see an adult smoking away in the front seat of their car, with their children in the back seat. They either don't care about, or don't understand, the negative consequences of this practice. With all the media reports regarding the negative effects of smoking, the former is more likely. The addiction to cigarettes is more powerful than the love they have for their family or friends.

ETS comes in two forms, sidestream smoke (smoke from the end of a lit cigarette, cigar, or pipe), and mainstream smoke (smoke exhaled by the smoker). This involuntary smoking, forced upon virtually everyone, exposes unwilling victims to the same superfluity of toxic, noxious, and harmful chemicals to which the smokers are exposed. Disappointingly, many smokers choose to smoke near playgrounds, schools, parks, and other locations frequented by children. As children play hard and breathe heavily, they become the unfortunate recipients of significant levels of ETS.

ETS is classified as a known human carcinogen by the Environmental Protection Agency (EPA), International Agency for Research on Cancer (IARC), a division of the World Health

Organization (WHO), and the United States National Toxicology Program[61]. ETS can linger in the air long after the source has been extinguished and can cause or exacerbate many adverse health effects, including cancer, respiratory infections, and asthma[62]. Exposure to ETS can ultimately lead to disease and death among those who do not smoke. In fact, ETS causes 3,400 lung cancer deaths and 46,000 heart disease deaths in nonsmokers in the United States each year[63]. This is an astounding fact, and it should give all of us reason to fight for greater rights for nonsmokers. Eliminating exposure to ETS and avoiding this assault should be a conscious effort for all of us. The best protection would be to ban tobacco products outright. Unfortunately, this is extremely unlikely to happen, so the next best thing would be to limit smoking to the smoker's place of residence. Again, this is not likely to happen, as the rights of the few seem to outweigh the rights of the majority with regard to this issue. Governments are willing to overlook this problem as they receive millions of dollars in cigarette taxes.

ETS is especially harmful to children under the age of eighteen months, among whom it is responsible for up to 300,000 lower respiratory infections, 15,000 hospitalizations, and 430 cases of sudden infant death syndrome each year[64]. Shamefully, 21 million children in the United States live in homes where they are exposed to ETS on a regular basis[65]. Should smokers then be held civilly and criminally responsible for these illnesses and deaths? Is this not a form of child abuse? These smokers are, in fact, willingly and knowingly exposing their children and the children of others to a harmful and sometimes deadly substance. How would a person be treated if they knowingly exposed their children to other toxic substances that resulted in injury or death? There simply is no safe or risk-free level of exposure to ETS. Each time you unwillingly inhale ETS, you are risking adverse health effects. The Surgeon General has reported that even short-term exposure to ETS can cause significant problems with blood vessels, blood platelets, and heart function, potentially increasing heart attack risk[66].

Lost productivity in the work place is another consequence of smoking. Not only do smokers take several breaks per day to smoke, they also tend to be less healthy and to require more sick time off than those who don't smoke. The Campaign for Tobacco Free Kids estimates annual productivity loss related to smoking in the United States to be $97.6 billion dollars per year. Smokers also experience decreased value of homes and vehicles, as well as greater costs for health and life insurance.

Some smokers quit smoking and instead use what they feel is a more "healthful" form of tobacco, smokeless tobacco, also known as chew. The truth is that smokeless tobacco products are not a safe or harmless substitute for cigarettes, cigars, or pipe smoking, and in fact are more harmful to your mouth. Smokeless tobacco is linked with oral and pancreatic cancer, leukoplakia (sores in the mouth that can lead to cancer), receding gums, bone loss around the roots of the teeth, teeth abrasions, teeth staining, and bad breath[67]. Smokeless tobacco still contains over twenty known carcinogens[68], and many other chemicals, including the addictive drug, nicotine, and very high levels of tobacco-specific nitrosamines[69]. The longer a person uses smokeless tobacco products, the more likely they are to have mouth problems, including leukoplakia. This is also a repulsive habit in appearance. The person has a distended appearance to the lips and must expel the chew at some point, often in a can, or worse, on the ground.

It is wise to leave the tobacco products to the uses that the Lord recommends, as a bruise healing herb, and for sick cattle. However, even then, it must be used with great caution and prudence. Tobacco appears to have medicinal properties for sick animals and has its place when used appropriately. Dr. Rulon Francis conducted experiments with rats and the healing affects of tobacco juice on deliberately inflicted bruises after Brigham Young University's athletic department returned from the Balkan Games in Yugoslavia with stories that trainers had used tobacco spray on basketball players' bruises. His study concluded that the rat group that was treated with the tobacco had twenty percent more healing cells than those rats treated with distilled water only[70].

Staying clear of this powerful and debilitating herb is vitally important to maintain health. The use of tobacco products among church members led the prophet Joseph Smith to inquire of the Lord regarding this practice. Through this inquiry, we received the Word of Wisdom and the Lord's definitive answer and guidance that tobacco is not for man. Tobacco products should be abstained from and are unquestionably harmful to the body. President George A. Smith said, "In my judgment, the use of tobacco, as little a thing as it seems to some men, has been the means of destroying their spiritual life, has been the means of driving from them the companionship of the Spirit of the Father, has alienated then from the society of good men and women, and has brought upon them disregard and reproach of the children that have been born to them..."[71]. Obviously, cigarette smoking has drastic affects on spiritual well-being as well as physical well-being.

Chapter 4

Doctrine and Covenants 89:10

"And again, verily I say unto you, all wholesome herbs God hath ordained for the constitution, nature, and use of man—"

This verse is particularly important to me because I believe it was an answer to prayer and ultimately changed my life. For many months, I had experienced significant back pain and finally decided to get it checked out by a doctor. My doctor and the findings of a subsequent specialist confirmed that I had a degenerative joint disease, ankylosing spondylitis (AS). After examination by a rheumatologist, I was prescribed the normal regimen of prescription medicines, namely prescription strength non-steroidal anti-inflammatory drugs (NSAIDs), muscle relaxers, and prescription painkillers. At first, it provided great relief from the pain I suffered in my lower back. I thought that I had seen the end of my problems, but, in reality, they had only just begun. I began experiencing a common side effect of NSAIDs, stomach discomfort. The stomach pains were so excruciating that I wondered which pain was worse, my back or stomach pain. This was discussed with my doctor and an additional prescription was offered, a drug to reduce production of acid in the stomach. This only brought temporary relief of the stomach pain I was feeling and, within a couple weeks, the stomach pain had returned. At this point, I felt that I needed to make a decision between my back pain or my stomach pain. In addition, my immune system seemed weaker. I was very susceptible to any illness to which I was exposed and my overall well-being felt reduced.

As trials and hardships often do, this ordeal made me turn to the Lord for help. I didn't want to live with the back pain, but knew I could not continue with the stomach pain either. As I pondered and prayed for guidance, the Word of Wisdom kept coming to mind. I read the Word of Wisdom more carefully than I have ever before and I was impressed that this part of verse ten was my answer; "all wholesome herbs God hath ordained for the constitution, nature, and use of man—". This led me to seek herbs for the two health conditions with which I was now dealing. I fortunately came upon research relating to deglycyrrhizinated licorice (DGL). This proven remedy for all kinds of stomach and intestinal ulcers did the trick. My stomach pain was relieved very quickly, and best of all, it was a permanent solution. The DGL repaired the damage that the NSAIDs had done to my stomach lining.

With my stomach pain relieved, I completed further research to find natural means for managing my AS. I moved forward with a conviction and belief in herbs and their healing power. I had faith and was sure there must also be an herb, or herbs, to help me with my back condition. After much research, I indeed found a combination of herbs and nutrients that have helped tremendously. I no longer take, nor need, the NSAIDs that created further health problems. I have been able to manage my illness better with herbs than with NSAIDs and muscle relaxers and without the severe side effects. Furthermore, my overall health and well-being have improved. I have increased immunity to illness and feel more vitality.

Some revealing words are contained within this scripture. One dictionary states that the medical meaning of constitution is "the physical makeup of the body; including its functions, metabolic processes, reactions to stimuli, and resistance to the attack of pathogenic organisms"[72]. Another dictionary defines constitution as "the physical makeup of the individual, especially with respect to health, strength, and appearance of the body; the structure, composition, physical makeup, or nature of something"[73]. We are told that man was formed from the dust of the earth, and man must have the "dust", or elements, of the earth replenished in the body repeatedly in order to avoid ill health. Our Father in heaven is telling us this when He used the word constitution. We need to understand that our bodies require elements from the earth to survive and the best way to get these elements is through plants.

The word herb refers to plants that are beneficial to and healthful for man. Plants store nutrients that they draw from the soil and the air, including vitamins and minerals. When we consume plants, we gain these nutrients and use them to build up our bodies. Plants and herbs can regulate the functions and metabolic processes of the body and, in fact, that is their intention. God put them on the earth for our benefit and this purpose.

Wholesome is also very important. Wholesome means healthy, completeness, the state of being whole. Every plant God has created contains its peak nutrients, including vitamins and minerals, in their whole form. This is the form God intends us to eat them, because in this state, we receive the most benefit from available nutrients. We must also distinguish between wholesome and harmful herbs. Marijuana is an herb, but it is not wholesome, and it therefore should be avoided. Herbal usage requires skill and study; it is best to consult a qualified practitioner before self-treatment.

Ordained is another key word. It means to establish or order by decree or law. All things upon this earth were created by God and work according to His laws and within His order. Being thus, plants will work according to God's purpose inside the human body. When eaten in their unadulterated form, plant foods will promote a healing effect from within and stimulate the proper function of vital organs and biological processes. All of this is completed in a safe and gentle manner. God has infinite wisdom and He has placed on earth all the nutrient-rich plants we need to stay healthy. I am convinced God has placed herbs for the benefit of all conditions and disease known to man on Earth.

Herbs have been used as far back as recorded history is kept, and in all likelihood started with Adam and Eve. A conversation between Adam and Eve and God is recorded in the bible as "And God said, Behold, I have given you every herb bearing seed, which is upon the face of all the earth, and every tree, in the which is the fruit of a tree yielding seed; to you shall be for meat" (Genesis 1:29). Similar accounts are recorded in Moses 2:29 and Abraham 4:29. Adam and Eve were given instruction to utilize the herbs and fruits of the trees available to them for their "meat". This includes use as both food and medicine. In Ezekiel 47:12 we read "and the fruit thereof shall be for meat and the leaves thereof for medicine". This is another acknowledgement of the importance of using herbs as our medicine. Many plant leaves are used in medicinal teas, ground up and encapsulated, or turned into a tincture.

Ancient civilizations relied upon herbs as medicine, food, perfume, disinfectants, and sometimes as currency. The

Egyptians, Chinese, Greeks, Romans, and other societies all knew of and used the medicinal power of herbs. Hippocrates, an early Greek physician before the time of Christ, developed a system of medicine utilizing herbs. The Nephites were another ancient civilization well versed in the use of herbs as medicine. In Alma 46:40, we read "And there were some who died with fevers, which at some seasons of the year were very frequent in the land—but not so much so with fevers, because of the excellent qualities of the many plants and roots which God had prepared to remove the cause of disease, to which men were subject by the nature of the climate--". Herbs were used to treat these fevers and "remove the cause of disease" among the Nephites. They knew the power of herbs and used them with great skill to benefit their people. I have wondered if ancient texts of the Nephites exist that describe their medicinal uses of herbs. Herbal medicine was also commonly used among the early saints. The Newel K. Whitney store was known to have stocked foodstuffs, textiles, household and hardware goods, books, and herbal medicines. Brigham Young wrote a letter to the Mormon Battalion that contained the following advice:

A letter from Brigham Young:

Camp of Israel, Omaha Nation
Cutler's Park

August 19th, 1846

To Captain Jefferson Hunt and the Captains, Officers, and Soldiers of the Mormon Battalion.

We have the opportunity of sending to Fort Leavenworth this morning by Dr. Reed a package of twenty-five letters, which we improve, with his word of counsel to you all: If you are sick, live by faith, and let the surgeon's medicine alone. If you want to live, using only such herbs and mild food as are at your disposal. If you give heed to this counsel, you will prosper; but if not, we cannot be responsible for the consequences. A hint to the wise is sufficient.

In behalf of the council,

Brigham Young, President[74]

Another discourse from Brigham Young affirms his belief in people being responsible for their own health and the health of their families, as well as the significance of herbs in this care. He said "It is God's mind and will that they [every father and mother] should know just what to do for them [their children] when they are sick. Instead of calling for a doctor, you should administer to them by the laying on of hands and anointing them with oil, and give them mild food and herbs and medicine that you understand"[75]. Parents have the primary responsibility for their children. This includes caring for them when sick as much as they have means and knowledge to do so.

Subsequent presidents of the church have also declared their belief in the healing power of herbs. In 1982, President Spencer W. Kimball stated "We should do all we can for ourselves first: dieting, resting, taking simple herbs known to be effective, and applying common sense, especially to minor trouble"[76]. Currently, pediatricians are overloaded with parents who bring their children to the doctor for simple ailments such as colds. The doctor may feel obligated to provide an antibiotic so the parents don't feel like the trip and their money was wasted. Unfortunately, this contributes to the development of disease-resistant bacteria, and perpetuates the myth that we have to take our children to the doctor for every simple ailment.

In fact, most acute ailments can be healed by the body alone if it is allowed the opportunity. This includes consuming only mild foods and drinking plenty of clean water. Herbs are used to stimulate biological processes within a person, thus allowing the body to heal itself. They enhance the body's innate and natural ability to heal. An example of this innate ability is a cut on your arm. If there is no foreign object in it and the cut is kept clean and free of bacteria, it will heal itself. On the other hand, if an herbal ointment of Aloe Vera or Calendula is applied, the wound healing process will be enhanced. Nothing can increase the speed of the healing process within the body greater than its capabilities. The body will only heal as fast as it is designed. However, herbs and other natural methods provide the optimal environment and nourishment for the speediest healing to take place.

Herbs are not synthetic chemicals, as are most modern medicines. Though many modern medicines originate from plants and herbs, they are in an adulterated form. Man takes the active constituent (the one that is active biochemically and appears to have the most substantial affect) of the plant and removes it from the hundreds of other constituents contained within the plant to use it as medicine. This is an unnatural state. Man, in his arrogance, removes the protective constituents that God intended in the whole form of the plant, thus increasing or causing negative side effects associated with the one "active" constituent. Herbs promote the natural functions of the body with the hundreds of biochemical constituents they contain. God is the creator of all herbs and no man can match His knowledge of chemistry and biology; thus, it is misleading to believe that we can create synthetic chemicals that will function better than the herbs God created.

Herbs are tremendously safe when used by a skilled herbalist, or one knowledgeable in the usage of herbs. It is incongruous that the U.S. Food and Drug Administration is so prone to censure the effectiveness and safety of herbs, while promoting prescription drugs as safe and effective. The FDA continues to censure scientific research regarding the efficacy and safety of herbs in favor of toxic drugs. A comparison of the safety of herbs versus prescription drugs establishes a clear picture. Prescription drugs are estimated to cause 106,000 deaths and an astonishing 2,216,000[77] serious adverse drug reactions annually in the United States. Compare these astounding statistics to that of herbs and dietary supplements. In a twenty-three year period, 1.6 million exposures were reported[78] to poison control. An exposure is defined as a call to the poison control center reporting actual or potential exposure to a substance. It is possible the exposure didn't even occur. In addition, the exposure does not indicate the person experienced any negative effects as a result of the exposure. Of these 1.6 million exposures, it was reported that 251,799[79] of these cases required hospitalization. In twenty-two years, only 230[80] deaths have been reported as a result of dietary supplements, or about 10 per year. I find it interesting that the author of a dietary supplement essay that include these figures decries this report when, by his own numbers, prescription drugs are almost nine times more likely to cause an adverse reaction, and over ten thousand times more likely to be fatal.

We have to ask ourselves why the FDA does little to protect the public from poisonous and deadly drugs, while devoting significant attention to "protecting" the public from safe herbs. It seems lately that, every month, there is another prescription drug, previously approved for use by the FDA, being pulled from the shelves because of adverse reactions and deaths associated with its proper use. Maybe the FDA should spend more time investigating and evaluating the real threat to the American public, prescription drugs.

It is ironic that despite the United States having one of the most sophisticated and technologically advanced systems of medicine in the world, it ranks last among industrialized nations in preventable deaths[81]. This is mostly because the U.S. health care system does not practice primary preventative medicine – it practices sick care. The U.S. medical system chooses to focus on early detection methods rather than primary preventative measures like diet and lifestyle factors. Medical students receive very few, if any, courses aimed at nutrition and lifestyle factors that contribute to disease. Instead they are indoctrinated in the "pill or surgery for every ill" myth. The American public in many ways demands this. We do not wish to change our lifestyles and diets in order to maintain or improve health. Instead, we ask for the newest surgery or pill to save us from our poor choices. We want, and our scientists and doctors seek, the "miracle" cure for cancer, arthritis, diabetes, etc… rather than learning to prevent these diseases.

Maybe this is because it is easier, or maybe it is due to the lack of education and information provided to the American public in this regard. If our physicians are not receiving this knowledge from the medical schools, how are they to teach others about it? Knowledge truly is power, and if we can empower the general public with more education, all will become healthier. Another study places the U.S. as forty-fifth among average life expectancy at birth[82]. Many of the countries above the U.S. maintain better diets and they integrate more natural therapies, including herbs, into their health care systems. These countries take a more proactive approach to health care, whereas the U.S. system is reactive. These countries also tend to have more active lifestyles, when compared to the inhabitants of the United States.

The U.S. healthcare system is also hesitant, or unwilling, to integrate natural healing methods. Other countries utilize herbs, nutrition, vitamins and minerals, and lifestyle factors as integrative and all-encompassing approaches to health care. Meanwhile, U.S. physicians continue to rely upon drugs and surgery almost exclusively. These options are far more invasive than those used by other countries. An example of this is St. Johns Wort, an herb often used in other countries to treat mild to moderate depression. It has proven effective in the treatment of mild to moderate depression with very few side effects. In fact, several recent studies suggest side effects occur in only one to three percent of patients taking this beneficial herb[83]. On the other hand, the monoamine oxidase inhibitor (MAOI) drugs that are predominantly used in the U.S. for the treatment of depression carry with them a superfluity of adverse side effects, including a higher rate of suicide among teenagers[84]. Fifty percent of patients that take MAOIs experience some kind of adverse reaction to the MAOIs. This means these patients are sixteen to fifty times more likely to experience a negative effect while taking MAOIs versus St John's Wort.

This unfortunate reality is largely due to the power and influence of the multi-billion dollar prescription drug manufacturers. They invest billions of dollars in advertising and in medical schools, and they shower doctors with gifts and incentives to push their products. In my opinion, these manufacturers are another group of "evil and conspiring men". They don't want to investigate the safety and effectiveness of herbs, nor to promote them as treatments, because they can't patent an herb that God manufactured. There simply aren't the same billions of dollars to be made in dietary supplements as there are in expensive drugs.

Now, this does not meant that every prescription drug is bad, or that herbs have a corner on the healing market, nor does it mean that modern medicine should be abolished. Herbs and natural treatments should be used as complements with modern medicine. There is not one system of health that has the complete answer to every human ailment and disease. What we do know is that there are safer alternatives to many prescription drugs and surgery currently being utilized by U.S. physicians. There are also times when a prescription drug is appropriate, for example during acute, life-threatening situations. Because herbs work with the body and stimulate the power within the body to heal, they act more slowly than do prescription drugs. It would therefore be unwise to wait for this action to take place during an acute, life-threatening situation. Technology to diagnose disease is also beneficial. A proper diagnosis is often key in determining the best course of action to take in regards to disease treatment. Many advances have also been made that go beyond the scope of herbal healing. All beneficial treatments should be combined and utilized in health care, with a preference for the least invasive, safest, and most effective treatments. U.S. physicians, and especially medical schools, would be wise to investigate more open-mindedly the complementary treatments that are less invasive and harmful to the American public.

Health care costs are growing at a deplorable rate in the U.S. Insurance costs have consistently risen at a much higher rate than has inflation, or wages for that matter. In 2005, health care expenditures rose by 6.9 percent, or twice that of inflation[85]. Many Americans are without health insurance, not because they choose not to carry it, but because they can't afford it. Nearly 47 million Americans are uninsured[86]. Healthcare spending is 4.3 times the amount spent on our national defense[87]. Healthcare spending equals about $6,700 per person, and amounted to two TRILLION dollars in 2005[88]. These costs and expenditures could be reduced with the integration of herbs and dietary supplements into the U.S. health care system.

Going back to our St. John's Wort/MAOI example; St. John's Wort is a fraction of the cost of MAOI drugs. This is but one example; there are many other supplements proven effective in managing disease that could be implemented at significant cost savings. Regretfully, this is unlikely to happen, as the deep pockets of the pharmaceutical companies would not be padded with herbs as they have been with prescription drugs. There simply is not the same financial incentive in herbs as there is in prescription drugs. Again, "conspiring men" care more about profit than they do the health of millions of Americans.

Our health care system is riddled with inefficiencies, unnecessary and excessive tests, excessive administrative fees, inflated prices, waste, and fraud. One must ask if the United States has the best health care system, or simply the most expensive. The statistics seem to agree with the latter. If more effective and safe natural remedies were utilized in the U.S., how much money could our health care system save? How many lives could be improved upon or saved? We may never know the answer to these questions.

Chapter 5

Doctrine & Covenants 89:11 & 16

"Every herb in the season thereof, and every fruit in the season thereof; all these to be used with prudence and thanksgiving.

All grain is good for the food of man; as also the fruit of the vine; that which yieldeth fruit, whether in the ground or above the ground-"

Fruits and vegetables should make up the bulk of the diet, particularly vegetables. We would be wise not to ignore the important health benefits of fruits and vegetables. Most fruits and vegetables are low in fat and calories and none contain cholesterol. They are high in potassium and fiber, both important nutrients to maintain a healthy body. Diets high in potassium may help control blood pressure and dietary fiber helps reduce cholesterol, reducing the risk of heart disease. Fiber is also important to maintain proper bowel function.

In order to take full advantage of the nutrients and phytochemicals contained in fruits and vegetables, eat a variety of colors. Each vegetable or fruit has its own make-up of beneficial vitamins, minerals, and other nutrients. These vitamins and minerals regulate body functions and facilitate chemical reactions within the body. It is best to add as much diversity as possible when eating fruits and vegetables, in order to gain the maximum benefit of their disease preventing phytonutrients. The skins of fruits and vegetables are particularly important because they hold many of these vital nutrients.

Vegetables provide the broadest range of phytochemicals, vitamins, and minerals of any food group. Dark green vegetables like spinach, broccoli, and romaine lettuce contain nutrients that are beneficial to the bones, lungs, immune system, and brain. Orange vegetables like carrots, pumpkin, and sweet potatoes promote eye health, help maintain blood sugar control, and contain cancer-fighting carotenoids. Starchy vegetables like potatoes and corn contain a unique blend of antioxidants and significant quantities of many vitamins and minerals. As you can see, the Lord, in His infinite wisdom, has made a multiplicity and abundance of vegetables, each with its own distinctive health benefits.

When fruits and vegetables are eaten in their unrefined, unprocessed, fresh, and natural state, a large proportion of the carbohydrates are "complex". Complex carbohydrates provide a significant amount of fiber, phytochemicals, vitamins, minerals, enzymes, and useable energy for the body. All of the nutrients that God intended us to receive are in these wholesome foods. Complex carbohydrates are digested more slowly, curtailing large swings in blood sugar. Keep in mind that the more you cook fruits or vegetables, the more nutrients and phytochemicals you destroy. Soaking vegetables in water removes some of the nutrients into the water and should be avoided, unless your intent is to drink the water as well. Overcooking also changes the flavor of vegetables.

Studies have found that those who eat the most fruits and vegetables as part of their regular diet have the lowest risk of coronary heart disease[89][90] and stroke[91]. In addition, the regular consumption of fruits and vegetables as part of a healthy diet may reduce the risk of type 2 diabetes and protect against certain cancers[92]. Because most vegetables are low in fat and calories, and none have cholesterol; when more of them that are eaten in place of high calorie, high fat, high cholesterol foods, more protection is afforded against obesity and other chronic illnesses. Most vegetables and fruits promote an alkaline blood environment. Alkaline blood is more resistant to disease and infection. Disease causing agents like bacteria and viruses require an acidic environment in which to thrive.

Most people should strive to include five to ten servings of fruits and vegetables in their daily diet. This may seem a daunting task at first, but it can be accomplishable with proper planning and an understanding of what equates a serving. A general guideline to follow is that the amount of fruits or vegetables you can fit into one half cup is a serving. The exceptions to this rule are lettuce and other leafy greens, where one full cup equals one serving, and dried fruit, which only requires one quarter cup to equal a serving. Fruits and vegetables should be included at every meal and in a wide assortment. Including a broad array stimulates the senses with a diversity of colors, smells, and tastes. No one fruit or vegetable contains all nutrients one needs, thus it is prudent to include many in the diet.

The high fiber content found in fruits and vegetables is beneficial to the gastrointestinal system and colon, and promotes regular function of the bowel. Because fiber is resistant to digestion, it soaks up water like a sponge as it passes through the digestive system and this speeds elimination. It also reduces pressure on the intestinal tract and may help prevent constipation, diverticuli (development of small, irritable pouches inside the colon), and diverticulitis (the painful inflammation of these pouches). High fiber foods provide a feeling of fullness with fewer calories. This may help reduce the overall caloric intake in your diet and reduce snacking. The natural water and sugar content in fruits and vegetables (especially fruits) speed metabolism and waste elimination, helping to cleanse the body of toxins and wastes.

Eye health is improved with the vitamins and phytochemicals found in vegetables. Vegetables high in vitamin A support night vision, and the carotenoids, lutein and zeaxanthin, have been shown to accumulate in the eye, providing protection to their sensitive tissues[93]. These carotenoids are found in abundance in dark green leafy vegetables and some fruits. When your mother told you to eat your carrots because it would promote healthy vision, she was right. Because of their high vitamin A and carotenoid content, a diet rich in fruits and vegetables may even protect against cataracts and macular degeneration.

Fruits and vegetables that are rich in potassium may help maintain healthy blood pressure[94]. In fact, increasing potassium may be more effective in lowering blood pressure than is decreasing sodium intake. Recent studies have shown that decreasing salt intake alone is less effective. Additionally, these fruits and vegetables may reduce the risk of developing kidney stones, and may help to decrease bone loss[95]. The electrolyte, potassium, regulates water balance within the body, as well as the acid-alkali balance in the blood and tissues. This mineral is very important to cellular function and helps to generate muscle contractions and it regulates the heartbeat. As with most vitamins and minerals, the best way to get this mineral is from your diet, which therefore requires a substantial intake of the proper fruits and vegetables.

Another important consideration is the body's acid alkali balance. The cells of the human body are swimming in a vast amount of liquid that is either acidic or alkaline. The blood should remain slightly alkaline or neutral to promote optimal health. Internal body functions operate best in a neutral to slightly alkaline environment, while disease thrives in an acidic environment. An alkaline environment is optimal for cellular and metabolic processes to occur. If the fluids of the body shift too far to the acid side, life and health sustaining biological and cellular processes fail to function properly. Too much acid in bodily fluids also reduces the ability to absorb vitamins and minerals, promotes toxic overload, and decreases immune system function. If this over-acidity begins to take place, the body will protect itself by buffering the acid with alkaline minerals (calcium, magnesium, potassium, and sodium) from the body's mineral reserves. When these reserves are depleted, the body borrows from whatever source it can find, including the bones and vital organs. If this process of borrowing continues for too long, the bones, muscles, and organs are weakened, and poor health can result.

Most experts recommend that between sixty-five and eighty percent of your diet should be alkaline. In fact, some research suggests that cancer cells thrive in an acidic environment and deteriorate in an alkaline environment. Your proper dietary intake will vary, depending on many factors. Supplying the body with the proper balance of alkaline and acid producing foods is very important to cellular and total health. The following is a short, but far from all-encompassing, list of common alkaline and acidic foods:

Common Alkaline Foods: Almonds, Apples, Apricots, Avocados, Bananas, Beans, Broccoli, Brazil Nuts, Cabbage, Carrots, Cauliflower, Celery, Cherries, Cucumbers, Grapes, Green beans, Lettuce, Mushrooms, Onions, Peaches, Pears, Potatoes, Raisins, Raspberries, Soy beans, Strawberries, Tomatoes, Watermelon

Common Acidic Foods: Bacon, Beef, Beer, Blueberries, Bread, Butter, Cashews, Cheese, Chicken, Chocolate, Coffee, Cola, Eggs, Ice Cream, Lamb, Lobster, Milk, Mustard, Oysters, Pasta, Peanuts, Peanut Butter, Peas, Pecans, Pork, Salmon, Sausage, Shrimp, Soft drinks, Sugar, Turkey, Walnuts.

The Lord gives us important direction when He says "in the season thereof". When we eat fruits and vegetables in season, we eat them at their peak nutrient levels. We get their full complement of vitamins, minerals, phytonutrients, enzymes, and fiber; all that God intended for us to receive from their consumption. It is best to eat locally grown produce whenever possible, because most produce that is not locally grown is picked before it is fully ripened (thus, not fully developed nutritionally), and then shipped to us often from hundreds of miles away. Some of this produce is irradiated during the journey to the grocery store to prevent spoilage and to eliminate harmful microorganisms, further depleting nutrients.

The most beneficial way to eat fruits is raw and vegetables raw or steamed. Eating them in this form leaves the majority of the beneficial nutrients intact. Steamed may be the optimal way to eat vegetables because it minimally reduces nutrient content while softening vegetables to make them more digestible. Cooking vegetables reduces their nutrient content, but too many raw vegetables in the diet can cause indigestion and gas.

Despite all of the arguments from non-organic farmers to the contrary, the healthiest produce is organic. Organic produce is not laced with chemical pesticides or waxes, nor is it irradiated (the process of exposing produce to radiation to disinfect, sanitize, and preserve produce). Even if you wash your produce, pesticides leach into the skins of the produce and you consume small quantities of these poisons each time you eat non-organic produce. If you compare an organic apple to a non-organic apple, the non-organic apple will be more esthetically appealing. This is due to the wax sprayed on the fruit to make it more attractive. Some fruits are even dyed to make them appear more lush and vibrant. This has nothing to do with taste, only appearance. You can't always judge a fruit by its cover. When you consume the two fruits, the organic apple is crisper and more flavorful. The phytonutrients found in fruits and vegetables provide the color, scent, and flavor in vegetables and work within the human body to promote health. They may even strengthen the immune system. Some studies maintain that citrus fruits have dozens of anti-cancer compounds alone. The powerful phytonutrients in fruits and vegetables are very beneficial in preventing disease, and for normalizing body function and chemistry.

The fruits and vegetables that come in certain seasons contain necessary phytonutrients for that particular season. God intends us to eat these plant foods in the season thereof, for us to receive maximum nutritional benefit. This doesn't mean that we can't consume fruits and vegetables out of their normal season, but it does indicate the superiority of nutrients obtained during their season. In spring, the earth is replenished after the cold of winter; plants grow and flourish, and Earth's full beauty radiates. During this season, we receive greens, vegetables, berries, and fruits to build our bodies back up after being somewhat dormant during the winter months. In the summer, we get melons, fruits, and vegetables that provide the necessary nutrients for our bodies to withstand the heat. Many of these fruits contain significant amounts of water, to quench our thirst during the heat of summer. The fall provides plant foods that enable our bodies to prepare for the cold winter ahead. Just before winter arrives, we are able to harvest a variety of foods that will store in a natural and nourishing state and are valuable for our winter diet. Winter is generally a period of less activity, requiring us to monitor more closely the foods we consume, in order to avoid putting on excess weight. The exceptions would be those people who live in very cold climates and who require extra nutrients to maintain proper body heat and insulation from the cold.

Chlorophyll is the basic component of a plant's blood. It is produced as a result of plants absorbing sunlight. When humans consume chlorophyll, it has a soothing effect on the mucous linings and helps in the detoxification process (particularly the liver). Applied topically, chlorophyll is beneficial for skin ulcers[96]. The lifeblood of plants, chlorophyll appears to have important healing and therapeutic effects on humans.

For a brief description of the primary nutrients (including vitamins, minerals, and phytonutrients) found in common fruits and vegetables, see appendix A. The nutrients are listed in alphabetical order, not in amounts of nutrients. While it is not a complete list of the nutrients that these plant foods contain, it does give a good overview of them. This chart is meant as a guide to help you determine what fruits and vegetables to include in your diet to ensure a well rounded range of nutrients. More information can be obtained from the U.S. Department of Agriculture Food and Nutrition Center website.

Hopefully, you will take the time to at least peruse the nutrients you are gaining or might be missing, based upon the common foods you consume. If not, make sure to look at this information later. With a basic idea of what nutrients are available from fruits and vegetables, it is important that you understand their function within the body. Appendix B is a summary of the function of the nutrients listed in appendix A. Additionally, the Dietary Reference Intake (DRI) established by the Food and Nutrition Board of the Institute of Medicine is listed. This value is established for a healthy adult, and is considered the amount sufficient to avoid deficiency disease. Please note that it doesn't consider the individual nature of human beings, nor optimal health. Your actual needs can, and will likely vary greatly from the DRIs.

If you reviewed both appendices, you can clearly see that the consumption of fruits and vegetables provides a multiplicity of health benefits. There would be less disease and better overall health for humankind if more fruits and vegetables were eaten in place of fatty high calorie foods. The health of many would be improved if we would snack on fruits and vegetables as a substitute for candy and junk food. It is also obvious that fruits and vegetables exert a powerful effect in the control, management, and reversal of diseases and adverse health conditions.

Chapter 6

Doctrine and Covenants 89:12-13

"Yea, flesh also of beasts and of the fowls of the air, I the Lord, have ordained for the use of man with thanksgiving; nevertheless they are to be used sparingly.

And it is pleasing unto me that they should not be used, only in time of winter, or of cold, or famine."

It is obvious that the Lord made animals available for our consumption. However, most people read the first portion of this verse indicating it is acceptable to consume animals without regarding the counsel to use them sparingly and in times of cold, winter, or famine. The fact is that the more animal products you consume, the greater your risk for disease. Adversely, the more plant foods you consume, the lesser your risk of disease. The average American consumes about eight ounces of meat per day, or over one hundred eighty pounds of meat per year[97]. This is significantly more than the two to three ounces per day recommended as part of a healthy diet. Americans who consume high quantities of meat are simply eating themselves to death.

Most of us grew up on this type of diet and many may not know how to cook a "meatless" meal. Many studies indicate that overconsumption of meat is associated with an increased risk for cancer, diabetes, asthma, arthritis, and heart disease. In fact, an epidemiological study demonstrated that pre-menopausal women who ate more than 3.7 ounces of meat per day increased their risk of breast cancer by twelve percent, while consumption below this threshold was associated with a thirty-two percent decrease in breast cancer risk[98]. Post-menopausal women fared even worse. Even when they consumed low levels of meat, the study indicated a fifty-two percent increase in breast cancer, and high levels of meat consumption increased risk by sixty-three percent[99]. Another study indicated that red meats and processed meats increased colorectal cancer rates up to thirty-five and forty-nine percent, respectively[100]. Red meat has also been associated with significantly elevated risk of esophageal, liver, and lung cancers[101]. That twelve-ounce steak we love to eat at restaurants may be contributing to debilitating diseases.

Red meat, processed meats, and pork are the worst meats for your health. Healthier meat choices are fish, seafood, turkey, and chicken. Of course, all of these choices can be made worse by the manner in which they are cooked. Frying and smoking meats increases the adverse health effects associated with meat. If you choose to include red meats in your diet, purchase lean cuts and try to limit consumption to three ounces of meat per day or less. The human gastrointestinal system is pocketed in design. This design, coupled with too much meat consumption, allows meat to putrefy and decompose in the intestines, promoting an ideal environment for bacteria and pathogens to develop.

Fat is often characterized as something we should avoid entirely in the diet. It has the reputation as the primary contributor to obesity. However, good fats perform many beneficial functions within the body. Fat is a useful source of energy – a more efficient source than protein. Fat plays a role in the absorption and utilization of the fat-soluble vitamins A, D, E, and K. Fat is a fundamental part of the membrane that surrounds each cell in the body. It also makes up the covering that protects nerve cells and is a structural component of cell membranes in the brain. Fatty acids promote healthy skin and regulate body temperature by nourishing the insulating layer of fat just below the skin. Vital organs, such as the kidneys and heart, are surrounded and protected by fat. Additionally, fat adds flavor and taste to food.

Moderate consumption of fat is healthy and necessary, particularly the right kinds of fat. However, too much fat is a contributing factor in degenerative diseases such as heart disease and diabetes. Moreover, the right type of fat is essential for the health of the body. The essential fatty acids, omega-3 and omega-6, are necessary for human health. They are considered essential because they can't be manufactured by the body. This means that you must obtain these important fatty acids from your food. Most Americans consume way too many omega-6 fatty acids compared to omega-3. A proper balance between these two acids is important to promote optimal health. A healthy diet includes a reduction in saturated fat, trans fat, and omega-6 fatty acids, combined with an increase in omega-3 fatty acids. It simply isn't enough to reduce unhealthy fats from the diet – they must be substituted for healthy fats.

Omega-3 fatty acids are divided into three major categories: alpha-linolenic acid (ALA), eicosapentaeonic acid (EPA), and docosahexaenoic acid (DHA). ALA is converted to DHA and EPA within the body. These oils are predominantly found in cold-water fish, some nut oils, and certain plants. The benefit of plant-based omega-3 fatty acids is that they generally also contain vitamin E to help prevent rancidity. Omega-3 fatty acids play a vital role in normal growth and development, as well as in brain function. Omega-3 fatty acids have been shown to reduce inflammation as well as the risk of many chronic diseases such as cancer, arthritis, and heart disease. They are highly concentrated within the brain and appear to be very important for brain and behavioral function. Deficiency in this fatty acid is a contributing factor in many illnesses.

Omega-6 fatty acids are found in meats and most vegetable oils. They work with omega-3 fatty acids to promote proper brain function, and normal growth and development. However, excess consumption of omega-6 fatty acids promotes inflammation, and increases risks of many chronic diseases. These should therefore be consumed sparingly.

Another type of fatty acids is omega-9, which isn't considered an essential fatty acid because the body can produce small amounts of it, as long as sufficient quantities of omega-3 and omega-6 fatty acids are present. Olive oil is the best source of omega-9, but it can also be obtained from avocados, almonds, sesame oil, cashews and more.

The kinds of fats that should be particularly avoided or limited are saturated fat, trans fat, or partially hydrogenated fats. Saturated fat is predominantly obtained from animal sources and is the main dietary cause of high blood cholesterol. Eating too much saturated fat increases the risk of heart disease by promoting the buildup of cholesterol within the arteries. Foods high in saturated fat also contain excessive calories, which further increases the chance of obesity. Saturated fat raises bad cholesterol (LDL) and decreases good cholesterol (HDL), thus increasing risk of stroke and atherosclerosis.

Trans fat, or partially hydrogenated fat, is a mostly man-made fat. It is naturally found in small amounts in beef, pork, lamb, and butterfat. It is manufactured by adding hydrogen to vegetable oil through a process called hydrogenation. One might ask why anyone would want to manufacture fat. The reason behind the manufacture of trans fat is that is has a longer shelf life and a better flavor stability than do other fats. In addition, it is inexpensive to produce, gives food a more desirable taste (addicting people to poor nutritional choices), and adds texture to foods. Just like saturated fats, trans fats raise blood cholesterol, perhaps at a greater rate than saturated fats. Trans fats raise LDL cholesterol and lower HDL cholesterol, increasing the risk of heart disease and stroke. Trans fats are commonly found in potato chips, fried foods, margarine, cookies, pies, and cakes. Recently, the government has required food labels to indicate the amount of trans fat that a food product contains.

The American Heart Association recommends that the amount of saturated fat in the diet be limited to seven percent, and trans fats to one percent of total daily calories. For a 2000-calorie diet, this equates to 140 calories from saturated fat and 20 calories from Trans fat, or 16 and 2 grams daily. To put this in perspective, a McDonald's quarter pounder with cheese contains 12 grams saturated fat and 1.5 grams trans fat, if you add an order of small fries, you add 1.5 additional grams of saturated fat[102]. If you choose a Burger King Whopper with cheese and small fries instead, you consume 19 grams saturated fat and 4.5 grams Trans fat[103]. Incredibly, both of these hamburgers contain more saturated fat than an eight ounce steak at Sizzler, which checks in at 11 grams saturated fat[104]. Fast food is virtually devoid of nutrients, but is packed with bad fats, refined sugar, and excessive calories. If you eat either of these meals mentioned above, you would have a difficult time eating two other meals that would not put your intake of bad fats significantly above what is considered healthy. If you do eat out, try to choose healthier alternatives. More restaurants are incorporating healthier options to their menu. Don't be afraid to ask for nutritional information also.

Protein is necessary for many body functions, as has been already mentioned. Animal products, including dairy, provide a significant amount of protein in the diet. Over-consumption of meat produces excess free radicals that damage the cells of the body. Again, people who eat the most animal-based foods tend to have the most chronic disease. A rodent-based study regarding cancer and protein intake yielded some interesting results. The rodents were dosed with the carcinogen aflatoxin, and then fed either a five percent or twenty percent protein diet. The rats fed the twenty percent protein diet had significantly higher levels of cancer, while most of those fed the five percent protein diet were cancer free[105]. This suggests that diet, particularly animal protein consumption, plays an important part in cancer initiation. The other interesting finding of this study was that rodents fed plant proteins, even at very high levels, did not experience the same level of cancer as those fed animal protein. In fact, plant based foods decreased tumor development. It appears that protein from animal sources provides the optimal environment to trigger cancer initiation and growth, while plant proteins do the opposite.

The protein used in this study was the milk protein casein. It is remarkable that human beings are the only mammal that continues to drink milk into adulthood. The fact is, milk promotes congestion in the body, depresses the immune system, and is associated with greater disease risk including diabetes, heart disease, and cancer. Because milk promotes clogging and mucus formation, it is associated with constipation, especially in children. Some studies have indicated that eliminating dairy products from children's diets reduced constipation. If this is a concern among your children, it may be worth a try to eliminate dairy foods for several days. Another concern with dairy products is that a significant percentage of the world population is lactose intolerant, meaning that they can't digest the milk sugar, lactose. We have all been told, and we grew up believing, that milk was a good source of calcium and that it strengthened bones. The Dairy Council uses celebrities with milk mustaches to promote drinking milk as a nutritious and healthy activity. The Dairy Council even went as far as to promote drinking milk as a beneficial weight loss measure. These misleading advertisements continued until research proved otherwise and the Dairy Council was forced to remove them.

The idea that drinking milk equates to strong bones is not completely accurate. While an eight-ounce serving of milk provides significant amounts of calcium, approximately 300 mg, only about one third of it is in an absorbable form. Furthermore, the process of pasteurization reduces calcium absorption rates even further. Pasteurization, which the FDA requires, is the process of heating milk or other liquids to a temperature that kills ninety plus percent of bacteria. This potentially leaves ten percent of the pathogenic bacteria in milk, while destroying the healthy bacteria as well.

Milk is made up of two protein molecules, casein (which is about eighty percent of milk protein) and whey protein. Casein is difficult to absorb and has been associated with cancer. A Harvard review suggests a positive association between high intake of dairy products and prostate cancer in men; an increase of fifty percent compared to those who consume minimal amounts of dairy products[106]. Whey, on the other hand, is high-quality and very absorbable complete protein, containing all of the essential amino acids.

Another dairy product, cheese, is loaded with salt as a preservative, and Americans love their cheese, putting it on almost anything. One dairy product that does have health-promoting effects is yogurt. Yogurt is an excellent source of healthy bacteria, or probiotics. Probiotics are healthy bacteria that inhabit the gut, leaving fewer places for harmful bacteria to attach. Because they occupy space in the gut, they help to avoid overgrowth of harmful bacteria. The challenge is to find yogurt that isn't loaded with sugar. Most commercially prepared yogurt is overloaded with sugar, almost to the point of overcoming the health-promoting benefits of consuming yogurt. It is better to make your own yogurt at home, or find a fat-free commercial product with reduced sugar.

There is wisdom in the last part of verse thirteen. The Lord is directing us to times when it is most acceptable, and in fact prudent, to consume meat. Before the advent of the refrigerator and freezer, fruits and vegetables could not be stored and kept for long periods of time. Our forefathers had to eat the fruits and vegetables "in the season thereof", and could not rely upon a freezer to keep them from spoiling, in order to consume them at a later date. Without freezers and refrigerators, they had to rely upon fresh meat to sustain life. They had to use animals as their source of food because it was the only food source available.

When famine occurs, it is generally because crops can't grow. There may be a drought and insufficient rain to produce crops of grain, or to grow vegetables or fruits. It may be the result of a natural disaster that destroys crops. When famine occurs, man must seek out whatever food he can obtain. This includes flesh of beasts and fowls of the air, though even animals can be scarce during famines when they too are fighting for scarce resources.

We have a superb example of the positive health effects of abstaining from meats in the first chapter of Daniel. In this chapter, we read the story of Daniel and other Hebrew children who are brought by Nebuchadnezzar, king of Babylon, into his court to be trained alongside the king's seed and the princes. These were children chosen because they had no blemish, were well favored, wise, skillful, and cunning in knowledge and understanding of science. Therefore, we could say that, from their description, they appear to be healthy, both physically and mentally, and on equal ground when they were brought into the king's court. As part of this three-year training process, Ashpenaz, the master of the eunuchs, was given charge to supply these children with a portion of the king's meat and wine. However, Daniel knew this was not the most nutritious diet and requested of Ashpenaz that he and other Hebrew children be allowed to eat pulse instead. Pulse is defined as foods made of seeds and grains. Ashpenaz did not want to disobey the king's orders and initially resisted. However, Daniel persuaded him to allow a ten-day trial of the pulse diet versus the traditional diet provided by the king and then determine which diet was better. Ashpenaz consented and the trial of diets began. After ten days, those who ate pulse appeared healthier than those who ate the portion of the king's meat and wine.

It is very interesting that a noticeable difference could be gained in only ten days. This is another testament to a predominantly plant food diet. In addition to appearing physically healthier, God blessed Daniel and the other children with "knowledge and skill in learning and wisdom". Proper nutrition does appear to correlate with mental capacity and health. Deficiencies in proper foods create deficiencies in the supply of nutrients to the brain. Foods can and do have a tremendous impact on mood and mental and emotional health. President Ezra Taft Benson said, "There is no question that the health of the body affects the spirit, or the Lord would never have revealed the Word of Wisdom. God has never given any temporal commandments—that which affects our bodies also affects our souls[107]."

Eating meat sparingly provides obvious enhanced physical health and even mental health, but there are additional environmental issues that are important to this subject as well. The majority of corn and soy grown in the world is used as livestock feed. This is food taken out of the mouths of children and adults, in order for the more affluent to gratify their desires for animal flesh. If those accustomed to the westernized diet consumed less meat, there would be less corn and soy required to feed cattle, pigs, and chickens; thus providing more food for the destitute and impoverished. This could make a significant impact in diminishing the tragic deaths from starvation and hunger each day. Cattle have stomachs predominantly meant to digest grass. The purpose of feeding cattle grain is to promote rapid weight gain, getting them to market more quickly. The larger the cow, the greater are the profits.

There is also the matter of pollution caused by livestock. According to the Environmental Protection Agency, nearly seventy-five percent of all water quality problems are agriculture related[108]. Much of current agriculture is conducted to feed the animals we consume. Inevitably, animal wastes, hormones and antibiotics given to livestock get into the water supply. This does not take into account the significant amounts of pesticides and chemical fertilizers that are used on crops fed to livestock. If this practice continues unchecked, it is possible that the water supply will deteriorate to an unsafe level for human consumption. Large quantities of water are withdrawn for the production of feed and for livestock to drink, again taking this precious resource away from humankind.

Livestock play a significant role in greenhouse gas emissions. In fact, the livestock sector generates more greenhouse gases, as measured in CO_2 equivalents, than does transportation[109]. Given all the vehicles on this earth, that is an astounding statistic. I would venture to say that the majority of people would believe that just the opposite is true. It is estimated that thirty percent of the earth's land surface is dedicated to raising livestock, and seventy percent of the former forests of the

Amazon have been turned over to grazing pastures[110]. This causes significant land degradation and water pollution. Moreover, animals that inhabit the rain forest, as well as important plants, are destroyed, all in the name of satisfying man's desire for meat.

This doesn't mean that you should abstain completely from meat and become a vegetarian. I am not advocating a strict vegetarian diet at all. The Lord has provided everything on this earth for the use of man and this includes animals. However, we must use prudence and exercise moderation when we consume the flesh of beasts and fowls of the air. Meat, in small quantities, is part of a healthy diet, but the key is small quantities. I doubt that the Lord intended 'sparingly' to be two meat meals a day, as is common in affluent societies. According to Merriam-Webster's dictionary, sparingly means "marked by or practicing careful restraint (as in the use of resources)". It is beneficial to have several meals per week without any meat included. Instead, substitute protein sources such as beans, lentils, soy foods, and whole grains. Reducing meat consumption increases health, and benefits the earth as well.

Chapter 7

Doctrine and Covenants 89:14-15 & 17

"All grain is ordained for the use of man and beasts, to be the staff of life, not only for man but for the beasts of the field, and the fowls of the heaven, and all wild animals that run and creep on the earth;

And these hath God made for use of man only in times of famine and excess hunger.

Nevertheless, wheat for man, and corn for the ox, and oats for the horse, and rye for the fowls and for swine, and all beasts of the field, and barley for useful animals, and for mild drinks, as also other grain."

Grains have been cultivated for their edible seeds and enjoyed for generations. Grains are the dietary staple for many cultures. Many years ago, our mothers would bake homemade bread. The smell of it was obvious upon entering our homes. The distinctive and delicious odor made your mouth water instantly. Today, those days are almost entirely gone. Very few people take the time to make homemade bread, and if they do have time, they probably don't have the knowledge. Instead, we consume empty calories from commercially prepared and refined white bread. This unfortunate event is taking a great toll on our health.

The grain refining process removes the bran and germ of grains and takes with it most of the fiber, vitamins and minerals. White flour is produced by refining and often bleaching whole wheat, destroying more than half of the nutrients wheat contains in its whole form. This includes vitamins B1, B2, B3, E, folic acid, calcium, zinc, iron, phosphorus, copper, and fiber. That is a long list of healthful nutrients being destroyed and removed from wheat. Wheat is thus placed in an unnatural, damaged, and less nourishing state – a form less nutrient dense than when God made it and in a state other than how He intended us to eat it. What God has created for man as food cannot be improved upon by man. In fact, generally when man alters food from its natural state, its nutritional value is reduced. President Benson stated "the more food we eat in its natural state—the less refined, and the fewer additives it contains—the healthier it will be for us".[111] Besides the better taste and aroma of homemade whole wheat bread, it is healthier.

Refined grains are milled and processed to "improve" their appearance and texture, increase their volume, and make them more stable for a longer shelf life. However, the outcome of this process is a considerable loss of nutrients. In fact, weevils generally prefer to infest whole wheat flour versus white flour, because the latter does not provide enough nutrients for their survival. If the weevil will die from refined white flour consumption, think about what it is doing to man. Manufacturers have tried to overcome the loss of nutrients that occurs by "enriching" refined grains. Using the word enriched for this process is erroneous, since the enrichment process only adds vitamins B1, B2, B3, and iron back to the processed grain. Other essential nutrients such as fiber, calcium, phosphorus, zinc, and folic acid are ignored. Enriching means to improve upon or enhance and the grain "enriching" process does neither of these when compared to wheat in its whole form.

Grains are called the staff of life because they have been so historically important for humankind's survival and have formed an essential part of our diet for thousands of years. Joseph of Egypt stored grains after interpreting the king of Egypt's dream about seven years of plenty followed by seven lean years. Grains store well for many years with minimal nutrient loss, especially when placed in proper containers and stored at proper temperatures. Whole grains are significant sources of fiber, potassium, iron, the B vitamins, selenium, magnesium, and other essential nutrients.

People who eat whole grains instead of refined grains achieve many health benefits, including reduced risk of chronic diseases such as coronary heart disease, atherosclerosis, stroke, obesity, and diabetes. You may be surprised to know that eating whole grains can help you control your weight. Increased consumption of whole grains is inversely associated with weight gain because of its high fiber content, which reduces constipation and water retention. On the other hand, the consumption of refined grains is associated with weight gain. We usually will eat larger portions of refined grains because they are not as satisfying as whole grains. This translates to the consumption of a greater quantity of empty calories.

Folate gained from whole grains is indispensible during pregnancy to prevent neural tube defects during fetal development. Without proper levels of folate, the developing fetus can experience significant retardation of proper growth. Whole grains also help reduce cholesterol due to their high fiber content. The B vitamins in whole grains play a role in metabolism by helping to release energy from the foods we consume. Magnesium, found in whole grains, helps to build strong bones and is a co-factor for enzymes involved in the body's use of glucose and in insulin secretion. Selenium, found in whole grains, is a powerful antioxidant, protecting cells form oxidative damage, and it helps to promote healthy immune system function.

Whole grains contain phytonutrients called lignans that act as weak hormone-like substances in the body. Lignans accelerate the metabolism of estrogen and occupy estrogen receptors in the body, helping to protect against breast cancer in women[112]. In fact, pre-menopausal women who eat greater than thirty grams of fiber per day reduce their risk of breast cancer by fifty percent[113]. Lignans also seem to benefit men because of their ability to bind to and precipitate testosterone, a hormone believed to increase prostate tumor growth[114]. Lignans are associated with lower incidence of cancer, diabetes, cardiovascular disease, and kidney disease.

The polyunsaturated fats, plant sterols, saponins, and oligosaccharides in whole grains have cholesterol-lowering effects. High cholesterol is something that afflicts many Americans and eating more whole grains could be of great benefit. You may have seen the many advertisements on oat cereals claiming this effect. Indeed, dietary factors are the most important element of a cholesterol management strategy. A small reduction in cholesterol can provide a significant protective effect against heart disease, the number one killer of Americans. Whole grains also have a significant quantity of antioxidants that protect cells against oxidative damage, including selenium and vitamin E. The phytoestrogens in whole grains not only occupy estrogen receptors, and bind to testosterone; they also can affect cholesterol levels and blood vessel elasticity. Thus, they promote the health of the cardiovascular system. Clinical trials have indicated that whole grains are associated with increased insulin sensitivity, one of the factors associated with type 2 diabetes. If more whole grains were consumed in the United States, fewer people would have to suffer with this miserable disease.

Whole grains are complex carbohydrates, meaning that during the digestive process, they are broken down in a controlled, regulated manner. This is in contrast to refined carbohydrates that provide a rush of energy because they are broken down so quickly. The bulk of carbohydrates in your diet should be complex. Simple carbohydrates, such as refined sugar and flour, result in increased caloric intake, and create nutrient deficiencies, as these foods are "empty calories" (high calorie and poor nutrition). When we are full of junk, we are less likely to eat foods that contain essential nutrients. Complex carbohydrates are also more satisfying as compared to simple carbohydrates, providing a feeling of fullness.

There are many different types of grain, each providing unique flavor, phytonutrients, and health benefits. Worldwide, wheat, corn, and rice make up the majority of grain production. Each culture is different in the type and quantity of grain consumed. In China and India, rice is the favorite grain, while here in the United States and Canada, wheat is the predominant grain. The grains discussed below are those most commonly consumed by man and/or named in this revelation.

Wheat

The Lord tells us all grains are provided for the use of man and beasts, but He further states that wheat is for man. Wheat is the most important cereal crop in the world, providing nourishment for more people than any other food. It appears, from the Lord's counsel, that we gain more nutritional value and benefit from wheat than any other grain on the earth. We may want to consider this the next time we are choosing between whole wheat and white bread. When you compare a slice of white bread versus wheat bread, the whole wheat slice has more than fifteen times the amount of vitamin E and three times as much fiber. Among the major grains, wheat has the highest protein content. President Ezra T. Benson stated "Most of us are acquainted with some of the prohibitions of the Word of Wisdom…..But what needs additional emphasis are the positive aspects – the need for vegetables, fruits, and grain, particularly wheat"[115].

Wheat is full of beneficial nutrients when in its natural and unrefined state, including fiber, manganese, vitamins B1, B2, B3, B5, B6, E, folic acid, calcium phosphorus, zinc, copper, protein, iron, and magnesium. It is used heavily for breads because of its gluten content. Gluten is a protein found in many grains, but in greatest quantities in wheat. It provides elasticity to bread and allows bakers to create satisfying risen bread.

The consumption of whole wheat products is associated with lower incidence of colon cancer, breast cancer, promotes regular bowel function, and reduces the risk of diverticular disease. This information supports the historical use of wheat bran as a bulk laxative. Some of the health benefits of wheat may be due to one of its metabolites called betaine. Betaine has the ability to reduce levels of inflammatory markers that are linked to a number of chronic conditions such as heart disease, diabetes, osteoporosis, and reduced cognitive function.

Wheat bran is an anti-cancer food. Interestingly, wheat bran has been shown to be beneficial in preventing colon cancer, whereas corn and oats have not shown the same effect[116]. It appears wheat has something extraordinary in it that other grains do not.

Wheat germ is a concentrated nutrient source, and contains high amounts of oil and vitamin E, which protects the oil from oxidizing too quickly. Vitamin E has healing properties of its own as a powerful antioxidant. Vitamin E helps reduce LDL cholesterol, is an essential nutrient for the immune system, and helps form red blood cells.

Rice

Rice is the second most consumed grain in the world. Over half of the world's population depends upon rice for food. It is particularly popular in Asia and India where it is used for most meals. In fact, the same word is used for rice and food in China. Unfortunately, just like wheat, most of the rice we consume is in an adulterated form. We seem to prefer white to brown when it comes to our grains. White rice has a more pleasing appearance, is easier for most people to digest, and is less chewy than brown rice. White rice is made by removing the germ and bran of brown rice, stripping it of important nutrients, and then polishing it into white rice. This milling and polishing process removes over sixty percent of the vitamins and minerals contained in brown rice. Brown rice is a good source of protein, vitamins B1, B2, B3, and B6, as well as the minerals phosphorus, iron, selenium, and manganese. In fact, one cup of brown rice supplies almost an entire days worth of the recommended daily allowance of manganese and over twenty-five percent of the RDA of selenium. Brown rice is lower in fiber than other grains, but it contains good quantities of essential amino acids. Brown rice is another food that would go a long way in the typical westernized diet if it were substituted for less nutritious white rice.

Corn

Corn is a versatile grain used both in fresh and dry form. It is widely cultivated in America and very popular in summer when the ears are ripe. Many farms are covered in the familiar appearance of corn stocks. We even turn these fields into mazes during the fall. Popcorn is low in calories and is a popular snack food. You can't watch a movie without popcorn, right? Unfortunately most corn is not grown for human consumption; rather, it is grown for livestock consumption or other products such as ethanol fuel, syrups, sweeteners, and oils. Corn provides respectable amounts of vitamins B1, B5, C, E, folic acid, and the minerals magnesium and phosphorus, as well as good amounts of fiber and essential fatty acids. However, it is not considered to be a complete food because people who rely heavily upon corn as a food source run the risk of pellagra. Pellagra is disease caused by a deficiency of niacin. The niacin content in corn is not very absorbable thus creating this risk. The Native Americans used corn as the staple in their diet but avoided pellagra by adding mineral ash to it when consumed. Corn is also low in protein, but is a good source of fiber. Corn contains very high levels of the antioxidants lycopene and vitamin C, which may slow disease progression. Indeed corn was found to have the greatest antioxidant activity among grains in one study[117]. Yellow corn, the most common corn used today, provides high levels of lutein, a carotenoid linked with protection against heart disease and macular degeneration. Next time you eat corn on the cob, forgo the butter and salt and taste the true flavor of corn. It won't take long before you wonder why you ever put butter and salt so heavily on your corn.

Oats

Oats are the fourth leading grain produced in the United States and are famous for their health benefits. Very little of total oat production is consumed by humans since most is fed to livestock. It is predominantly used as a breakfast cereal, like oatmeal. Oatmeal is an excellent and healthy choice for breakfast because it provides sustained energy. It is digested slowly and methodically rather than quickly like other breakfast cereals. For those who are sensitive to wheat, oat bran is a good substitute. Oat flour can be used in both bread and cookies.

Oats are hulled for consumption, but this does not remove the bran and germ, leaving the nutrients intact. Oats have good quantities of selenium, magnesium, phosphorous, manganese, and iron, as well as fiber and vitamin B1. Oats contain a high percentage of complex carbohydrates, which help reduce the risk of certain cancers, diabetes, and bowel irregularity. Oats are famous for their ability to reduce the risk of heart disease and many cereals manufactured from oats put this claim on their box. Oats also contain an excellent amino acid profile, as well as balanced amounts of essential fatty acids and they provide many essential proteins necessary for optimum functioning of the body. Compared to other grains, oats contain high levels of unsaturated fat in the germ. Oats reduce blood glucose and insulin responses, which is essential in preventing diabetes complications. This helps control blood glucose swings associated with diabetes. A polysaccharide in oats, beta-glucan, may enhance immune system function, and lower cholesterol levels. Many studies have demonstrated significant reduction of high cholesterol levels is possible with frequent oat consumption. Oats also contain, avenanthramides, antioxidants that help protect the blood vessels from LDL cholesterol damage.

Barley

Barley has a rich flavor similar to nuts and is used as a sweetener as well as to manufacture alcoholic products. Barley is a hardy grain and grows well in cold climates. Most barley is fed to livestock. Barley has a very similar nutritional makeup to corn but it contains good quantities of niacin and high levels of fiber and selenium. The fiber in barley, like oats, is high in beta-glucan, which helps lower cholesterol and reduces the risk of heart disease. Barley drinks have been used medicinally for many years.

Rye

Rye has an appearance similar to that of wheat. It is very hardy, growing in inhospitable soil and in cold climates. Rye can be used without other grains to produce pleasing leavened bread. Bread produced from rye is more dense and heavier than bread produced from wheat. It has a lower glycemic index than most grains and is therefore beneficial to diabetics. The type of fiber in rye promotes a prompt feeling of fullness, making it an ideal grain to consume when trying to lose weight. Rye is an excellent source of manganese and selenium, and provides good levels of phosphorous, magnesium, and protein.

Chapter 8

Doctrine and Covenants 89:18-21

"And all saints who remember to keep and do these sayings, walking in obedience to the commandments, shall receive health in their navel and marrow in their bones;

And shall find wisdom and great reassures of knowledge, even hidden treasures; And shall run and not be weary, and shall walk and not faint.

And I, the Lord, give them a promise, that the destroying angel shall pass by them, as the children of Israel, and not slay them. Amen. "

God wants us to have joy and happiness. One of the conditions for us to realize this joy and happiness is obedience to His law of health. Members of the Church of Jesus Christ of Latter Day Saints commit to following the Word of Wisdom, which entails so much more than abstaining from tea and coffee. The Word of Wisdom includes avoidance of all harmful substances, but more importantly teaches us of that which is beneficial and nourishing to the body. Obedience to the Word of Wisdom is a matter of personal worthiness to members of the church. After all, blessings are predicated on obedience, and obedience means we are willing to submit our will to the Father's. The Lord created and gave us miraculous physical bodies and He expects us to take proper care of them. Those who live the Word of Wisdom to its fullest will generally live longer and more worthwhile lives. President Gordon B. Hinckley said, "I give thanks to our Creator for revealing unto His prophet what we call the Word of Wisdom. I do not hesitate to say that in this brief but inclusive statement of the Lord is found counsel, given with a promise, which, if more widely observed, would save untold pain and suffering and lead not only to increased physical well-being but also to great and satisfying "treasures of knowledge" of the things of God.[118]"

There is too much disease and premature death and too few very healthy people in the world today. The Word of Wisdom has never been needed more than it is now. Obedience to this revelation will bring greater health and vitality, and ultimately a greater quality of life, not just quantity. This doesn't mean that you will be disease free or avoid death. It means you will achieve your personal optimum level of health. You will be able to live your life to the fullest extent, gaining the fullest experiences necessary for you to progress in God's eternal plan. Your body will be fortified with a greater resistance to disease and illness and your immune system will be stronger. This doesn't mean you will avoid death or disease, as these are both part of mortal life. Death is a necessary step toward the next realm of existence and disease is often necessary to strengthen and try us. If we never experience sickness and pain, we will not fully appreciate health and pleasure.

With better health comes a realized decrease in health expenditures. As you take care of your body and avoid harmful substances, you will spend less on "sick" care and prevent wasteful expenditure on harmful substances. Imagine what you could save if you currently fill your thirty-two ounce mug twice daily or more with soda and replace it with water. The savings of someone who currently smokes goes beyond just the cost of a pack of cigarettes. The health care savings of quitting smoking will be immeasurable in the long run. Additionally, you will preclude yourself from enduring the difficult process of overcoming addiction.

Addiction is very challenging and problematic to overcome. It requires a strong conviction and desire to quit, coupled with the support of family, friends, health professionals, and wise leaders. If you have already succumbed to addiction, I urge you to begin the process back to physical and spiritual health now. As you eliminate and overcome your addiction, you will see measurable improvements in your health and well-being. The process of overcoming addiction will be challenging and you will face many struggles, but it will be well worth it. You will replace temporary pleasure with true joy. You may not be successful at first, but you can beat the addiction if you have the desire to do so and receive the necessary help. Don't forget to plead for help from the Lord. Above all, don't feel unworthy to speak to Him. He is anxious to help you. He waits with open arms and outstretched hands willing to listen to you and give you all the help you need. He will not leave you alone to complete this task if you ask for His help.

The Word of Wisdom is not just for the physical body. Obedience to the Word of Wisdom also promises increased wisdom, knowledge, and spiritual power. Disobedience to it will result in damage to spiritual growth and a decreased capacity to avoid other detrimental practices. Wisdom is the proper use of knowledge. The Word of Wisdom provides knowledge and those who live its precepts are exercising wisdom. President Joseph Fielding Smith said, "The truth is that spiritual salvation is dependent upon the temporal far more than most men realize. The line of demarcation between the temporal, or physical, and the spiritual, cannot be definitely seen. The Lord has said that he has not given a temporal commandment at any time. To men, some of these commandments may be temporal, but they are spiritual to the Lord because they all have a bearing on the spiritual, or eternal, welfare of mankind.[119]"

It is obvious that how we treat the physical body directly correlates with our spiritual health. When we have an active, healthy body, our inner spiritual strength can grow and thrive. Optimum physical health affords maximum mental capacity. We have a greater capacity to learn and think clearly, when our physical bodies are healthy. With this greater capacity will come the "hidden treasures of knowledge" the Lord promises.

The Word of Wisdom is simple and practical, but does not spell out everything that we should and should not consume. The Lord will not "command in all things" nor provide a detailed list for us to follow. The Lord expects us to use prudence and wisdom and to exercise personal judgment based upon the guidance in this revelation. Again quoting President Joseph Fielding Smith, "Such revelation is unnecessary. The Word of Wisdom is a basic law. It points the way and gives us ample instruction in regard to both food and drink, good for the body and also detrimental. If we sincerely follow what is written with the aid of the Spirit of the Lord, we need no further counsel…Thus, by keeping the commandments, we are promised inspiration and the guidance of the Spirit of the Lord, through which we will know what is good and what is bad for the body[120]". Prayerful and thoughtful consideration is necessary because each one of us has different needs. We are all biologically different. As we follow the Lord's counsel and seek personal inspiration, the Lord will guide us to the best foods for us individually and for our families.

While the Word of Wisdom does not need scientific evidence to back it up, much of current scientific research lends credence to its principles and truthfulness. Looking at life expectancy for members of the Church of Jesus Christ of Latter Day Saints compared to non-members reveals a greater life expectancy. Male members of the church live an average of 7.3 years longer than non-member men while women live an average of 5.8 years longer than non-member women[121]. Cancer research also supports the Word of Wisdom. Male and female members of the church have a twenty-four percent lower incidence of all cancers as compared to non-members living in Utah[122]. It appears that proper dietary habits are more important than is location.

I testify that the Word of Wisdom was given to the prophet Joseph Smith directly from the Lord. It is meant for our benefit, for us to gain the best health and well-being possible. Obedience to the counsel contained therein will bring blessings to those who follow it, both temporal and spiritual. With obedience greater physical health, more self-control, greater clarity of mind, and more spiritual power will be realized. You will gain a closer relationship with your Heavenly Father and His Son Jesus Christ. I urge all of us to carefully examine what we take into our bodies and to make the necessary changes to gain all the blessings and rewards our Father in Heaven is waiting anxiously to provide.

APPENDIX A

FRUITS			
Fruit	**Vitamins**	**Minerals**	**Phytonutrients & Other Nutrients**
Apple (raw-with skin, 1 cup, quartered)	Folate (4 mcg) Vitamin A (68 IU) Vitamin C (5.7 mg) Vitamin E (.23 mg)	Calcium (7 mg) Potassium (134 mg) Phosphorus (14 mg) Magnesium (6 mg)	Fiber (2.9 mg) Pectin Quercetin
Apricot (raw, 1 cup, halved)	Vitamin A (2985 IU) Vitamin C (15.5 mg)	Calcium (21 mg) Iron (.6 mg) Potassium (402 mg)	Beta-carotene (1695 mcg) Lutein Protein (2.17 g) Quercetin
Avocado (raw, 1 cup, cubed)	Folate (122 mcg) Niacin (2.6 mg) Pantothenic Acid (2.1 mg) Vitamin A (219 IU) Vitamin B1 (.1 mg) Vitamin B2 (.2 mg) Vitamin B6 (.39 mg) Vitamin C (15 mg)	Calcium (18 mg) Iron (.82 mg) Magnesium (43 mg) Phosphorus (79 mg) Potassium (728 mg) Sodium (10 mg)	Alpha-carotene (36.09 mcg) Beta-carotene (92.37 mcg) Cryptoxanthin Fiber (10 g) Lutein Protein (2.99 g) Quercetin
Banana (raw, 1 cup, sliced)	Folate (30 mcg) Niacin (1 mg) Pantothenic Acid (.5 mg) Vitamin A (96 IU) Vitamin B6 (.55 mg) Vitamin C (13.1 mg) Vitamin E (.15 mg)	Calcium (8 mg) Iron (.38 mg) Magnesium Phosphorus (32 mg) Potassium (537 mg) Selenium (1.5 mcg)	Alpha-carotene (39.05 mcg) Beta-carotene (37.41 mcg) Fiber (5.7 g) Lutein Protein (1.64 g) Rutin
Blackberry (raw, 1 cup)	Folate (9 mcg) Vitamin A (80 IU) Vitamin C (14.4 mg) Vitamin E(.84 mg)	Calcium Iron (.41 mg) Magnesium (9 mg) Manganese (.08 mg) Phosphorus (18 mg) Potassium (114 mg) Selenium (.2 mcg) Zinc (.23 mg)	Epicatechin Fiber (3.6 g) Protein (2.0 g) Quercetin
Cantaloupe (raw, 1 cup, balls)	Folate (38 mcg) Vitamin A (5985 IU) Vitamin B6 (.13 mg) Vitamin C (65 mg)	Calcium (17 mg) Magnesium (21 mg) Phosphorus (27 mg) Potassium (473 mg)	Beta-carotene (3575.74 IU) Fiber (1.6 g) Protein (1.48 g) Rutin
Cherry (sweet, raw, 1 cup, without pits)	Vitamin A (98 IU) Vitamin C (10.8 mg)	Calcium (20 mg) Copper (.08 mg) Iron (.55 mg) Magnesium (17 mg) Manganese (.11 mg) Phosphorus (33 mg) Potassium (341 mg)	Anthocyanins Epicatechin
Cranberry (raw, 1 cup, whole)	Vitamin A (60 IU) Vitamin C (13.3 mg)	Calcium (8 mg) Phosphorus (13 mg) Potassium (85 mg) Selenium (.1 mcg)	Catechin Epicatechin Quercetin
Grape (raw, red or green, seedless, 1 cup)	Folate (3 mcg) Niacin (.28 mg) Vitamin A (100 IU) Vitamin C (16.3 mg)	Calcium (16 mg) Magnesium (11 mg) Phosphorus (31 mg) Potassium (289 mg)	Beta-carotene (59.52 mg) Protein (1.08 g) Resveratrol Saponins Quercetin

Grapefruit (raw, white, 1 cup, sections, with juice)	Vitamin C (76.6 mg) Vitamin A (75 IU)	Calcium (28 mg) Magnesium (21 mg) Phosphorus (18 mg) Potassium (340 mg)	Fiber (2.5 g) Limonoids Lycopene Pectin Protein (1.59 g)
Kiwi (raw, 1 cup)	Folate (44 mcg) Niacin (.6 mg) Vitamin A (154 IU) Vitamin B2 (.05 mg) Vitamin B6 (.11 mg) Vitamin C (164.1 mg) Vitamin E (2.58 mg)	Calcium (60 mg) Copper (.23 mg) Iron (.55 mg) Magnesium (29 mg) Phosphorus (60 mg) Potassium (552 mg) Selenium (.4 mcg) Zinc (.24 mg)	Beta-carotene (92.83 mg) Cryptoxanthin Fiber (5.4 g) Lutein Protein (2.02 g) Quercetin Zeaxanthin
Lemon (raw, without peel, 1 cup)	Vitamin A (48 IU) Vitamin C (112.4 mg)	Calcium (55 mg) Iron (1.27 mg) Magnesium (17 mg) Phosphorus (34 mg) Potassium (293 mg)	Coumarins Fiber (5.9 g) Limonene Protein (2.33 g)
Lime (raw, one fruit)	Folate (5 mg) Vitamin A (33 IU) Vitamin C (19.5 mg)	Calcium (22 mg) Iron (.4 mg) Magnesium (4 mg) Phosphorus (12 mg) Potassium (68 mg)	Coumarins Fiber (1.9 g)
Mango (raw, 1 cup, sliced)	Folate (23 mg) Niacin (.96 mg) Vitamin A (1262 IU) Vitamin B2 (.09 mg) Vitamin B6 (.22 mg) Vitamin C (45.7 mg) Vitamin E (1.85 mg)	Calcium (17 mg) Magnesium (15 mg) Phosphorus (18 mg) Potassium (257 mg) Selenium (1 mcg)	Catechin Fiber (3.0 g) Limonene Quercetin
Olive (raw, 1 cup, ripe, canned, small-extra large)	Vitamin A (544 IU) Vitamin E (2.24 mg)	Calcium (112 mg) Iron (4.48 mg) Selenium (1.6 mcg) Sodium (1168 mg)	Beta-carotene (3792 IU) Cryptoxanthin
Orange (raw, 1 cup, sections)	Folate (55 mg) Pantothenic Acid (.45 mg) Vitamin A (404 IU) Vitamin B1 (.16 mg) Vitamin C (95.8 mg)	Calcium (72 mg) Magnesium (18 mg) Phosphorus (25 mg) Potassium (326 mg) Selenium (.9 mcg)	Beta-carotene (127.93 IU) Fiber (4.3 g) Hesperidin Limonene Protein (1.69 g) Quercetin
Peach (raw, 1 cup, slices,	Folate (5 mg) Niacin (1.24 mg) Vitamin A (501 IU) Vitamin C (10.2 mg)	Calcium (9 mg) Magnesium (13 mg) Phosphorus (31 mg) Potassium (293 mg) Selenium (.1 mg)	Catechin Fiber (2.3 g) Protein (1.41 g) Quercetin
Pear (raw, 1 small fruit)	Folate (11 mg) Vitamin A (34 IU) Vitamin C (6.2 mg)	Calcium (14 mg) Manganese (.07 mg) Potassium (176 mg) Selenium (.1 mcg)	Fiber (4.5 g) Catechin Epicatechin Quercetin
Pineapple (raw, 1 cup, chunks, traditional variety)	Folate (17 mg) Niacin (.78 mg) Vitamin A (86 IU) Vitamin C (27.9 mg)	Calcium (21 mg) Magnesium (21 mg) Manganese (2.63 mg) Potassium (206 mg) Selenium (.1 mcg)	Beta-carotene (51.56 IU) Bromelain Fiber (2.3 g)
Plum (raw, 1 cup, sliced)	Vitamin A (570 IU) Vitamin C (15.7 mg)	Calcium (10 mg) Potassium (258 mg)	Catechin Epicatechin Fiber (2.3 g) Protein (1.16 g) Quercetin

Raspberry (raw, 1 cup)	Folate (26 mg) Niacin (.74 mg) Vitamin C (32.2 mg)	Calcium (31 mg) Iron (.85 mg) Magnesium (27 mg) Potassium (186 mg)	Fiber (8.0 g) Protein (1.47 g) Quercetin Selenium (.3 mcg)
Strawberry (raw, 1 cup, halves)	Folate (37 mg) Vitamin A (18 IU) Vitamin C (89.3 mg)	Calcium Magnesium (19 mg) Phosphorus (37 mg) Potassium (233 mg) Selenium (.6 mcg)	Fiber Fiber (3 g) Protein (1.01 g) Quercetin
Watermelon (raw, 1 cup, balls)	Folate (4 mg) Niacin (.28 mg) Vitamin A (877 IU) Vitamin B1 (.05 mg) Vitamin B6 (.07 mg) Vitamin C (12.5 mg)	Calcium (11 mg) Iron (.36 mg) Magnesium (15 mg) Phosphorus (18 mg) Potassium (173 mg) Selenium (.6 mg)	Beta-carotene (466.39 mg) Lutein Lycopene

VEGETABLES			
Vegetable	**Vitamins**	**Minerals**	**Phytonutrients & Nutrients**
Beet (Cooked, boiled, drained, sliced, no salt, 1 cup)	Folate (136 mg) Niacin (.56 mg) Vitamin A (58 mg)	Calcium (28 mg) Copper (.13 mg) Iron (1.34 mg) Magnesium (40 mg) Manganese (.55 mg) Phosphorus (64 mg) Potassium (518 mg)	Fiber (1.7 g) Protein (1.43 g) Quercetin
Broccoli (cooked, boiled, drained, no salt, small stalk-about 5" long)	Folate (151 mg) Vitamin A (2167 IU) Vitamin C (90.9 mg)	Calcium (56 mg) Iron (.94 mg) Magnesium (29 mg) Phosphorus (94 mg) Potassium (410 mg)	Fiber (4.7 g) Lutein Protein (3.33 g) Zeaxanthin
Cabbage (cooked, boiled, drained, no salt, 100 grams of edible portion)	Folate (22 mg) Vitamin C (1.7 mg)	Selenium (1.0 mcg)	Chlorophyll Lutein Quercetin
Carrot (baby, raw, 85 g)	Vitamin A (586 IU) Vitamin C (2.2 mg)	Calcium (27 mg) Iron (.76 mg) Magnesium (9 mg) Selenium (.7 mg)	Alpha-carotene (3201.53 IU) Beta-carotene (5432.35 IU) Coumarins Fiber (2.5 g) Lutein Lycopene Quercetin
Cauliflower (Cooked, boiled, drained, without salt, 1 cup)	Folate (54 mg) Vitamin C (55 mg)	Calcium (20 mg) Magnesium (12 mg) Potassium (176 mg) Selenium (.8 mcg)	Beta-sitosterol Fiber (2.8 g) Protein (2.28 g) Quercetin
Celery (raw, 1 cup, chopped)	Folate (36 mg) Vitamin A (454 IU) Vitamin C (3.1 mg)	Calcium (41 mg) Iodine Iron (.2 mg) Magnesium (11 mg) Potassium (263 mg) Zinc (.13 mg)	Coumarin Fiber (1.6 g) Quercetin Rutin
Corn (sweet, yellow,	Folate (48 mg) Niacin (1.66 mg)	Magnesium (27 mg) Phosphorus (77 mg)	Beta-carotene (67.82 IU) Fiber (2.9 g)

boiled, drained, no salt, 1 medium ear-about 7" long)	Vitamin A (271 mg)	Potassium (219 mg) Selenium (.2 mg)	Protein (3.42 g)
Cucumber (raw, peeled, sliced, 1 cup)	Folate (17 mg) Vitamin A (86 IU) Vitamin C (3.8 mg)	Calcium (17 mg) Iron (.27 mg) Magnesium(14 mg) Potassium (162 mg)	Beta-carotene (36.44 mg) Beta-sitosterol
Green Beans (raw, snap, 1 cup)	Folate (22 mg) Vitamin A (71 IU) Vitamin K (6.8 mcg)	Calcium (18 mg) Iron (.61 mg) Magnesium (9 mg) Selenium (.3 mcg)	Beta-carotene (63 IU)
Lettuce (green leaf, raw, 2 cups, shredded)	Folate (28 mg) Vitamin A (5332 IU) Vitamin C (13 mg)	Calcium (26 mg) Iron (.62 mg) Potassium (140 mg) Selenium (.4 mcg)	Chlorophyll Fiber (1 g) Lutein Pectin
Onion (raw, sliced, 1 cup)	Folate (21 mg) Vitamin C (8.5 mg)	Calcium (26 mg) Iron (.24 mg) Magnesium (11 mg) Selenium (.5 mg) Zinc (.19 mg)	Fiber (2.0 g) Protein (1.26 g) Quercetin Rutin Saponins
Pea (green, cooked, boiled, drained, no salt, 1 cup)	Folate (101 mg) Vitamin A (1282 IU) Vitamin C (22.7 mg) Vitamin E (.22 mg)	Calcium (43 mg) Iron (2.46 mg) Magnesium (62 mg) Phosphorus (187 mg) Potassium (434 mg)	Alpha-carotene (35.44 IU) Beta-carotene (751.42 IU) Fiber (8.8 mg) Lutein Protein (8.58 mg)
Pepper (sweet, green, raw, sliced, 1 cup)	Folate (10 mg) Niacin (.44 mg) Vitamin A (340 IU) Vitamin C (74 mg)	Calcium (9 mg) Iron (.31 mg) Potassium (261 mg)	Alpha-carotene (18.9 IU) Beta-carotene (191.73 IU) Bioflavonoids Fiber (1.5 g) Lutein Quercetin
Potato (baked, with skin, no salt, 1 medium)	Folate (48 mg) Niacin (2.44 mg) Pantothenic Acid (.65 mg) Vitamin B1 (.11 mg) Vitamin C (16.6 mg)	Calcium (26 mg) Iron (1.88 mg) Magnesium (49 mg) Manganese (.38 mg) Phosphorus (120 mg) Potassium (925 mg) Zinc (.61 mg)	Fiber (3.8 g) Lutein Protein (4.32 g) Quercetin Rutin
Pumpkin (pie mix, canned, 1 cup)	Niacin (1.01 mg) Pantothenic Acid (3.07 mg) Vitamin A (22405 IU) Vitamin C (9.5 mg)	Calcium (100 mg) Iron (2.86 mg) Magnesium (43 mg) Phosphorus (122 mg) Potassium (373 mg) Sodium (562 mg)	Beta-carotene Cryptoxanthin Fiber (22.4 g) Lutein Protein (2.94 g) Quercetin Zeaxanthin
Radish (raw, slices, 1 cup)	Folate (28 mg) Vitamin C (17.2 mg)	Calcium (29 mg) Iron (.39 mg) Selenium (.7 mg) Zinc (.33 mcg)	Fiber (1.9 g)
Spinach (raw, 2 cups)	Folate (116 mg) Niacin (.43 mg) Vitamin A (5626 IU) Vitamin C (16.8 mg)	Calcium (60 mg) Copper (.08 mg) Iron (1.6 mg) Magnesium (48 mg) Manganese (.54 mg) Potassium (334 mg) Zinc (.32 mg)	Beta-carotene (3375.8 IU) Fiber (1.4 g) Lutein Protein (1.72 g) Zeaxanthin
Squash (summer, all	Folate (36 mg) Vitamin A (381 IU)	Calcium (49 mg) Iron (.65 mg)	Beta-carotene (228.61 IU) Fiber (2.5 g)

varieties, cooked, boiled, drained, no salt, 1 cup, slices)	Vitamin C (9.9 mg)	Magnesium (43 mg) Phosphorus (70 mg) Potassium (346 mg) Selenium (.4 mcg)	Pectin Protein (1.64 g)
Sweet Potato (cooked, baked in skin, without salt, 1 medium-5" long"	Niacin (1.7 mg) Pantothenic Acid (1 mg) Vitamin A (21909 IU) Vitamin C (22.3 mg)	Calcium (43 mg) Iron (.79 mg) Potassium (542 mg) Selenium (.2 mcg) Zinc (.36 mg)	Alpha-carotene (49.5 IU) Beta-carotene (13120.65 IU) Fiber (3.8 g) Pectin Protein (2.29 g)
Tomato (red, ripe, raw, year-round average, 1 cup, chopped or sliced)	Folate (27 mg) Niacin (1.07 mg) Vitamin A (1500 IU) Vitamin B6 (.14 mg) Vitamin C (22.8 mg)	Calcium (18 mg) Iron (.49 mg) Magnesium (20 mg) Phosphorus (43 mg) Potassium (426 mg) Sodium (8 mg)	Beta-carotene (808.85 IU) Fiber (2.2 g) Lycopene Protein (1.59 g) Quercetin
Yam (cooked, boiled or baked, no salt, 1 cup, cubes)	Folate (22 mg) Vitamin A (165 IU) Vitamin C (16.5 mg)	Calcium (19 mg) Iron (.71 mg) Magnesium (24 mg) Potassium (911 mg) Selenium (1.0 mcg)	Fiber (5.3 g) Protein (2.03 g)

U.S. Department of Agriculture, Agricultural Research Service. 2002. USDA National Nutrient Database for Standard Reference, Release 15. Nutrient Data Laboratory Home Page, http://www.nal.usda.gov/fnic/foodcomp

APPENDIX B

Vitamin/ Mineral	DRI (Dietary Reference Intake)	Function/Purpose
Vitamin A	3000 IU	✓ Helps maintain hair, bones, and teeth ✓ Essential for eyes and skin ✓ Promotes proper immune system function
Vitamin B1 (Thiamin)	1.2 mg	✓ Necessary for carbohydrate metabolism ✓ Necessary for muscle coordination ✓ Promotes healthy nerve function
Vitamin B2 (Riboflavin)	1.8 mg	✓ Necessary for food metabolism and energy production ✓ Makes Vitamin B6 active in the body ✓ Beneficial for proper tissue repair
Vitamin B3 (Niacin)	16 mg	✓ Necessary to obtain energy from food ✓ Helps break down and use energy from carbohydrates, proteins, and fats ✓ Promotes health nerve function ✓ Promotes proper gastrointestinal system function ✓ Helps maintain healthy skin
Vitamin B5 (Pantotheni c Acid)	5 mg	✓ Helps the glands produce hormones and chemicals that regulate nerve function ✓ Helps create new fats and proteins in the body
Vitamin B6 (Pyridoxine)	1.7 mg	✓ Necessary for protein metabolism and absorption ✓ Necessary for carbohydrate metabolism ✓ Promotes nerve and brain function ✓ Plays a role in many enzymatic reactions within the body
Vitamin B12 (Cyano-cobalimin)	2 mcg	✓ Promotes normal nerve function ✓ Promotes normal blood function ✓ Helps from red blood cells

Folate (Folic Acid)	400 mg	✓ Helps prevent birth defects during pregnancy ✓ Essential for red blood cell formation ✓ Essential for protein metabolism
Vitamin C	90 mg	✓ Helps prevent oxidative damage ✓ Helps bind cells together ✓ Helps strengthen blood vessels ✓ Aids in the absorption of iron and copper ✓ Helps form collagen ✓ Helps regenerate and stabilize other vitamins ✓ Important for proper growth and repair of all body tissues ✓ Beneficial to the immune system
Vitamin D	400 IU	✓ Helps absorb calcium and phosphorus ✓ Helps build and maintain strong teeth and bones
Vitamin E	15 mg	✓ Helps prevent oxidative damage ✓ Helps form red blood cells ✓ Helps form muscles and other tissues ✓ Beneficial to the immune system ✓ Helps maintain cellular integrity
Vitamin K	120 mcg	✓ Necessary for normal blood clotting
Calcium	1300 mg	✓ Necessary for the development and maintenance of bones and teeth ✓ Promotes proper muscle and nerve function ✓ Helps activate enzymes necessary to convert food to energy ✓ Beneficial to cardiovascular health ✓ Helps blood clot
Copper	.9 mg	✓ Helps several enzymes function properly ✓ Helps form connective tissue ✓ Helps iron absorption ✓ Necessary to form red blood cells ✓ Important in the production of collagen, cartilage, bone, and connective tissue

Iron	18 mg	✓ Essential to form hemoglobin (the substance in blood that carries oxygen to the cells of the body)
Magnesium	420 mg	✓ Activates enzymes needed to release energy in the body ✓ Helps regulate potassium levels ✓ Essential for healthy bones and teeth ✓ Helps the muscles relax
Manganese	2.3 mg	✓ Essential for healthy bones and cartilage ✓ Necessary for normal tendon structure ✓ Helps facilitate metabolism of carbohydrates, fats, and protein
Phosphorus	1250 mg	✓ Helps build bones and teeth ✓ Necessary for metabolism of fats, proteins, and carbohydrates ✓ Helps maintain proper urine and blood acid/base balance
Potassium	N/A	✓ Helps the muscles contract ✓ Helps maintain regular fluid balance ✓ Necessary for nerve and muscle function
Selenium	55 mcg	✓ Helps prevent oxidative damage
Sodium	N/A	✓ Helps maintain water balance throughout the body ✓ Essential for nerve impulses
Zinc	11 mg	✓ Essential for normal growth and development ✓ Beneficial to the immune system ✓ Necessary for many enzymatic reactions that aid digestion and metabolism ✓ Stimulates wound and burn healing

Bromelain is an anti-inflammatory, proteolytic enzyme from pineapples. It aids the body in the digestion of protein, can help break down excess mucus in the respiratory system, and is a potent anti-inflammatory agent.

Beta-sitosterol is a phytosterol (plant compounds similar to cholesterol and steroid hormones). It limits cholesterol absorption within the body by blocking absorption sites. It has also been studied for its immune enhancing effects as well as for its anti-cancer properties[123].

Carotenoids (alpha-carotene, beta-carotene, cryptoxanthin, lycopene, and lutein) are the source of plants orange, yellow, and red colors. They are potent antioxidants, meaning that they help prevent oxidation of cells. Alpha-carotene, beta-carotene, and beta-cryptoxanthin convert to retinol (Vitamin A) in the body without the risk of toxicity. The conversion of these carotenoids to retinol decreases when the body's stores of Vitamin A are high. The antioxidant ability of carotenoids has been associated with decreased risk of certain cancers[124].

Chlorophyll is the plant's primary mechanism of photosynthesis (the process of transforming sunlight into fuel for cells). It gives plants their green color and is the primary component of plant's blood. The list of health promoting benefits from chlorophyll is long: it provides nourishment to the intestines, soothes the mucous linings, and detoxifies and purifies the body[125]. In addition, it has antioxidant, anti-inflammatory, and wound healing properties, and removes carbon dioxide and carbon monoxide from the body.

Coumarins are suspected of blocking the carcinogenic effects of chemicals and toxins. They have anti-tumor properties and stimulate the immune system and the enzyme responsible for anti-carcinogenic properties.

Flavonoids (anthocyanin, bioflavonoids, catechin, epicatechin, hesperidin, quercetin, and rutin) are antioxidant nutrients that provide color and flavor to the plants. These plant compounds provide protective benefits to plants, such as repairing damage and shielding the plant from toxins. Flavonoids are in large supply in fruits and vegetables. There are a large number of flavonoids, each of which provides its own list of health benefits including anti-tumor, immune enhancing, and antioxidant effects. Flavonoids work synergistically with, and increase the effectiveness of, vitamin C.

Fiber plays the important role of speeding the body's elimination process. Insoluble fiber, found in whole grains, is indigestible, adding bulk to digestive materials, speeding its movement through the digestive tract. This prevents toxins that have been sent for elimination from staying in the body, reducing the risk of disease and gallstones. Soluble fiber, found in fruits, vegetables, beans, legumes, seeds, oats, and barley, helps eliminate cholesterol and bile acids, which provides a protective benefit to the cardiovascular system. Adequate intake of fiber reduces constipation and can help prevent diverticular disease.

Limonoids exert anti fungal, anti-cancer, antiviral, and bactericidal effects. They have shown the ability to prevent the initiation of cancer and prevent the growth of certain tumors and cancers.[126]

Pectin, a soluble fiber mostly found in apples and citrus fruits has the potential to lower cholesterol, improve insulin resistance, relieve diarrhea, and it stimulates the immune system. Pectin promotes a feeling of fullness, possibly reducing overeating.

Resveratrol inhibits the initiation, promotion, and progression of cancer. It is a superb antioxidant and promotes cardiovascular health by lowering LDL cholesterol and reducing plaque buildup in the arteries.

Protein is an important part of cell function and the building blocks of any living organism. It is utilized to make enzymes, hormones, and other body chemicals. It is necessary for healthy nails and hair, as well as to build and repair tissues. Protein is essential for growth and maintenance.

Saponins are predominantly found in legumes and soy products. They bind to cholesterol, helping to remove it from the body. In addition, they may exert anti-cancer and anti-inflammatory properties. Saponins can also boost immune system activity, particularly the activity of interferon and T-lymphocytes. Research has indicated that saponins have anti tumor properties and the ability to kill cancer cells[127].

Index

References

[1] Skeel S, *What if no one were fat, retrieved April 30, 2008, from www.articles.moneycentral.msn.com/Insurance/Advice?WhatIfNoOneWere Fat.aspx?*

[2] Hinckley G, *Joseph Smith Jr. – Prophet of God, mighty servant,* Ensign, Dec 2005, 2-6.

[3] American Institute for Cancer Research, www.aicr.org, retrieved April 3, 2008.

[4] Center for Disease Control, www.cdc.gov/nchs/FASTATS/lcod.htm, retrieved April 3, 2008.

[5] Kant AK, Graubard B., Schatzkin A., *Dietary patterns predict mortality in national cohort.* The national health interview surveys, 1987 and 1992. Journal of Nutrition 134:1793-1799, 2004.

[6] Campbell TC, Campbell TM, *The China study,* Benbella Books 2004 p. 24.

[7] Center for Disease Control, www.cdc.gov/hchs/data/ad/ad381.pdf, retrieved April 8, 2008.

[8] Karvonen M, Pitkanieni J, Tuomilehto J. *The onset age of type 1 diabetes in Finnish children has become younger.* Diabetes Care 1999; 22; 1066-1070.

[9] Schoenle EJ, Lang-Muritano M, Gschwend S, et al. *Epidemiology of type 1 diabetes mellitus in Switzerland: steep rise in incidence in under 5 year old children in the past decade.* Diabetologica 2001; 44: 286-289.

[10] The Associated Press, *Skip the whole milk. Pass on soda. Drink Beer?* March 2006.

[11] Lesser LI,Ebbeling CB,Goozner M,Wypij D,Ludwig DS PLoS Medicine Vol. 4, No. 1, e5 doi:10.1371/journal.pmed.0040005.

[12] Diethelm PA, Rielle JC, McKee M, *The whole truth and nothing but the truth? The research Phillip Morris did not want you to see,* Lancet, Vol. 364 No. 9446, 2004.

[13] Smith JF, Conference report, October 1913, p. 14.

[14] Center for Disease Control, *Alcohol-attributable deaths and years of potential life lost – United States,* 2001, retrieved from www.cdc.gov/MMWR/preview/mmwrhtml/mm5337a2.htm#tab, April 16, 2008.

[15] Center for Disease Control, *Alcohol-attributable deaths and years of potential life lost – United States,* 2001, retrieved from

www.cdc.gov/MMWR/preview/mmwrhtml/mm5337a2.htm#tab, April 16, 2008.
[16] Reinberg S, *Even in middle age, starting drink may lower heart risks,* retrieved April 7, 2008, from www.businessweek.com/print/lifestyle/content/healthday/613342.html
[17] Boyles S, *Wine, fat intake linked to breast cancer*, retrieved April 7, 2008, from www.webmd.com/breast-cancer/news/20040317/wine-fat-intake-breast-cancer
[18] Murray, M et. al. *The condensed encyclopedia of healing foods.* Pocket Books Publishing 2006.
[19] Blaylock, R, *Health and nutrition secrets that can save your life.* Health Press 2006 p. 17.
[20] American Heart Association, *Alcohol wine and cardiovascular disease.* Retrieved April 7, 2008 from www.americanheartassociation.org.
[21] Smith J, as quoted by Joel H. Johnson, *A voice from the mountains,* Salt Lake City: Juvenile Instructor Office, 1881, p.12.
[22] Young B, *Discourses of Brigham Young selected and arranged by John A. Widstoe,* p. 182.
[23] Ludlow V, *Principles and practices of the restored gospel,* p. 434.
[24] Peterson H, *Q&A: questions and answers*, New Era, Oct. 1975, p. 36-37.
[25] Page L, *Healthy healing,* Healthy Healing Inc. 2006, p. 123.
[26] Haas E, Levin B, *Staying healthy with nutrition,* Celestial Arts Publishing, 2006.
[27] Stratton C, *Questions and answers,* Tambuli, Aug. 1980, p. 8.
[28] Rossignol AM, Bonnlander H, *Prevalence and severity of the premenstrual syndrome. Effects of foods and beverages that are sweet or high in sugar content,* Journal of Reproductive Medicine 36:131-36, 1991.
[29] Creighton SM, Stanton SL, *Caffeine: does it affect your bladder?,* British Journal of Urology 66(6):613-14, 1990.
[30] www.scorecard.org/chemical-profiles/summary.tcl?edf_substance_id=83-067-0#hazards , retrieved April 15, 2008.
[31] Journal of Clinical Nutrition 2001, March; 73(3):532-8.
[32] Environmental Protection Agency, www.epa.gov/ogwdw/hfacts.html, retrieved April 15, 2008.

---

[33] Page L, *Healthy healing,* Healthy Healing Inc. 2006, p. 592.
[34]
www.findarticles.com/p/articles/mi_m0876/is_n56/ai_9164614, retrieved April 16, 2008.
[35] Kaslow J, *Health issues associated with coffee and caffeine,* retrieved from http://www.drkaslow.com/html/coffee-caffeine.html, April 16, 2008.
[36] Haas E, Levin B, *Staying healthy with nutrition,* 2006.
[37] California Air Resources Board, *List of known ETS constituents.*
[38] World Health Organization, International Agency for Research on Cancer, June 2003.
[39] American Cancer Society, *Cigarette Smoking,* retrieved April 17, 2008, from
www.cancer.org/docroot/PED/content/PED_10_2X_Cigarette_Smoking.asp?sitearea=PED.
[40] U.S. Department of Health and Human Services, *Reducing the health consequences of smoking: 25 years of progress. A report of the surgeon general.* 1989.
[41] American Cancer Society, *Cigarette Smoking,* retrieved April 17, 2008, from
www.cancer.org/docroot/PED/content/PED_10_2X_Cigarette_Smoking.asp?sitearea=PED
[42] Government of Saskatchewan, *What are the health risks faced by tobacco users?,* retrieved April 17, 2008, from
www.health.gov.sk.ca/health-effects-tobacco.
[43] American Cancer Society, *Cigarette Smoking,* retrieved April 17, 2008, from
www.cancer.org/docroot/PED/content/PED_10_2X_Cigarette_Smoking.asp?sitearea=PED
[44] Environmental Protection Agency, retrieved April 18, 2008, from www.epa.gov/safewater/dwh/c-soc/benzopyr.html.
[45] Occupational Safety Hazard Association, *Cadmium*, retrieved October 28, 2008 from
www.osha.gov/SLTC/cadmium/index.html.
[46] http://quitsmoking.about.com/od/chemicalsmoke/p/TSNAs.htm, retrieved April 18, 2008.
[47] American Cancer Society, *Cigarette Smoking,* retrieved April 17, 2008, from

www.cancer.org/docroot/PED/content/PED_10_2X_Cigarette_Smoking.asp?sitearea=PED

[48] Connolly G, Alpert H, Wayne G, Koh H, *Trends in smoke nicotine yield and relationship to design characteristics among popular cigarette brands,* Harvard School of Public Health 2007.

[49] Environmental Protection Agency, retrieved April 18, 2008, from www.epa.gov/iaq/co.html#sources%20of%20Carbon%20Monoxide.

[50] Environmental Protection Agency, retrieved April 18, 2008, from www.epa.gov/iaq/co.html#sources%20of%20Carbon%20Monoxide.

[51] Occupational Safety Hazard Association, retrieved April 18, 2008, from www.osha.gov/dts/chemicalsampling/data/CH_218300.html.

[52] Environmental Protection Agency, retrieved April 18, 2008, from www.epa.gov/ttn/atw/hlthef/arsenic.html.

[53] Environmental Protection Agency, retrieved April 18, 2008, from www.epa.gov/ttn/atw/hlthef/benzene.html.

[54] Environmental Protection Agency, retrieved April 18, 2008, from www.epa.gov/minimize/factshts/cadmium.pdf.

[55] Environmental Protection Agency, retrieved April 18, 2008, from www.epa.gov/minimize/factshts/cadmium.pdf

[56] Environmental Protection Agency, retrieved April 18, 2008, from www.epa.gov/ttn/atw/hlthef/chlorofo.html.

[57] Environmental Protection Agency, retrieved April 18, 2008, from www.epa.gov/iris/subst/0419.htm.

[58] Environmental Protection Agency, retrieved April 18, 2008, from www.epa.gov/iris/subst/0419.htm.

[59] Environmental Protection Agency, retrieved April 22, 2008, from www.epa.gov/lead/pubs/leadinfo.htm.

[60] Environmental Protection Agency, retrieved April 18, 2008, from www.epa.gov/ttn/atw/hlthef/vinylchl.html.

[61] American Cancer Society, *Secondhand Smoke,* retrieved April 22, 2008, from http://www.cancer.org/docroot/PED/content/PED_10_2X_Secondhand_Smoke-Clean_Indoor_Air.asp.

[62] California Environmental Protection Agency, *Identification of environmental tobacco smoke as a toxic air contaminant,* Executive Summary, June 2005.

[63] California Environmental Protection Agency, *Identification of environmental tobacco smoke as a toxic air contaminant,* Executive Summary, June 2005.

[64] California Environmental Protection Agency, *Identification of environmental tobacco smoke as a toxic air contaminant,* Executive Summary, June 2005.

[65] Schuster MA, Franke T, Pham CB, *Smoking patterns of household members and visitors in homes with children in the United States,* Archives of Pediatric Adolescent Medicine, Vol. 156, 2002: 1094-1100.

[66] Surgeon General, U.S. Department of Health and Human Services, *The health consequences of involuntary exposure to tobacco smoke: 6 major conclusions of the surgeon general report,* 2006, retrieved April 22, 2008, from http://www.surgeongeneral.gov/library/secondhandsmoke/factsheets/factsheet6.html.

[67] American Cancer Society, *Smokeless tobacco and how to quit,* retrieved April 17, 2008, from http://www.cancer.org/docroot/PED_10_13X_Quitting_Smokeless_Tobacco.asp?sitearea=PED.

[68] National Caner Institute, *Smokeless tobacco and cancer: questions and answers,* retrieved April 17, 2008, from www.cancer.gov/cancertopics/factsheet/tobacco/smokeless.

[69] American Cancer Society, *Smokeless tobacco and how to quit,* retrieved April 17, 2008, from http://www.cancer.org/docroot/PED_10_13X_Quitting_Smokeless_Tobacco.asp?sitearea=PED.

[70] Science Watch, *No help for the hungry,* April 28, 1981, retrieved April 22, 2008, from http://query.nytimes.com/gst/fullpage.html?sec=technology&res=9B07E3DA1638F93BA15757C0A967948260.

[71] Smith G, Conference Report. 1918, p.40.

[72] http://medical-dictionary.thefreedictionary.com/constitution , retrieved April 23, 2008.

[73] www.meriam-webster.com/dictionary/constitution, retrieved April 23, 2008.

[74] Young B, Church Library, Journal History: August 19th, 1846, Salt Lake City.
[75] Young B, as reported by David W. Evans, *Discourse by President Brigham Young,* August 13, 1875.
[76] Kimball S, *President Kimball speaks out on administration to the sick,* Tambuli, August 1982, 34.
[77] Lazarou J, Pomeranz B, Corey PN, *Incidence of adverse drug reactions in hospitalized patients. A meta-analysis of prospective studies,* Journal of the American Medical Association 1998;279:1200-1205.
[78] Hurley D, *Diet supplements and safety: some disquieting data,* New York Times, January 16, 2007, corrected article February 6, 2007.
[79] Hurley D, *Diet supplements and safety: some disquieting data,* New York Times, January 16, 2007, corrected article February 6, 2007.
[80] Hurley D, *Diet supplements and safety: some disquieting data,* New York Times, January 16, 2007, corrected article February 6, 2007.
[81] Nolte E, McKee C, *Measuring the health of nations,* Health Affairs, January/February 2008, 27(1):58-71.
[82] Central Intelligence Agency, *The world fact book 2008, rank order of life expectancy at birth.*
[83] Mayo Clinic, retrieved April 25, 2008, from www.mayoclinic.com/health/st-johns-wort/NS_patient-stjohnswort
[84] Mayo Clinic, retrieved April 25, 2008, from www.mayoclinic.com/health/maois/MH00072
[85] Catlin A, Cowan C, Heffler S, et al, *National health spending in 2005,* Health Affairs 26:1 (2006): 142-153.
[86] California Health Care Foundation, *Health care costs 101 – 2005,* March 2, 2005, retrieved April 25, 2008, from www.chcf.org.
[87] California Health Care Foundation, *Health care costs 101 – 2005,* March 2, 2005, retrieved April 25, 2008, from www.chcf.org.
[88] Catlin A, Cowan C, Heffler S, et al, *National health spending in 2005,* Health Affairs 26:1 (2006): 142-153.
[89] He F, Nowson C, Lucas M, MacGregor G, *Increased consumption of fruits and vegetables is related to a reduced risk of coronary heart disease: meta-analysis of cohort studies,* J Hum Hypertens. 2007;21:717-28.
[90] Keys A, *Seven countries: a multivariate analysis of death and coronary heart disease,* London: Harvard University Press, 1980.

[91] He F, Nowson C, Mcgregor G, *Fruit and vegetable consumption and stroke: meta-analysis of cohort studies,* Lancet 2006;367:320-26.
[92] U.S. Department of Agriculture, *Why is it important to eat vegetables,* retrieved April 30, 2008, from www.mypyramid.gov/pyramid/vegetables_why.html.
[93] Krinsky N, Landrum J, Bone R, *Biological mechanisms of the protective role of lutein and zeaxanthin in the eye,* Annu Rev Nutr. 2003; 23:171-201.
[94] [94] U.S. Department of Agriculture, *Why is it important to eat vegetables,* retrieved April 30, 2008, from www.mypyramid.gov/pyramid/vegetables_why.html.
[95] [95] U.S. Department of Agriculture, *Why is it important to eat vegetables,* retrieved April 30, 2008, from www.mypyramid.gov/pyramid/vegetables_why.html.
[96] Haas E, Levin B, *Staying healthy with nutrition,* Celestial Arts Publishing, 2006.
[97] Bittman, M, *Rethinking the meat-guzzler. New York Times 2008.*
[98] Taylor, E, et al. *Meat consumption and risk of breast cancer in the UK women's cohort study.* British Journal of Cancer 2007;96:1139-1146.
[99] Taylor, E, et al. *Meat consumption and risk of breast cancer in the UK women's cohort study.* British Journal of Cancer 2007;96:1139-1146.
[100] Genkinger, J & Koushik, A. *Meat consumption and cancer risk.* PLoS Med 4(12): e345 doi:10.1371/journal.pmed.0040345.
[101] Genkinger J & Koushik A. *Meat consumption and cancer risk.* PLoS Med 4(12): e345 doi:10.1371/journal.pmed.0040345.
[102] www.nutirion.mcdonalds.com/bagamcmeal/nutrition_facts.html, retrieved October 16, 2008.
[103] www.bk.com, retrieved October 16, 2008.
[104] www.thedailyplate.com, retrieved October 16, 2008.
[105] Campbell T, Campbell T II, *The China study.* Benbella Books 2004.
[106] Chan J, Giocannucci E. *Dairy products, calcium, and vitamin D and the risk of prostate cancer.* Epidemiology Revs. 23 (2001): 87-92.
[107]Benson E, *In His steps.* Ensign, Sep 1988, 2.
[108] FAO report, *Livestock's long shadow - environmental issues and options.* Retrieved October 15, 2008 from www.fao.org/newsroom/en/news/2006/1000448/index.html.

---

[109] FAO report, *Livestock's long shadow - environmental issues and options.* Retrieved October 15, 2008 from www.fao.org/newsroom/en/news/2006/1000448/index.html.
[110] FAO report, *Livestock's long shadow - environmental issues and options.* Retrieved October 15, 2008 from www.fao.org/newsroom/en/news/2006/1000448/index.html.
[111] Benson E, *Do not despair.* Tambuli, March 1987, 2.
[112] www.whfoods.com. Retrieved October 22, 2008.
[113] www.whfoods.com. Retrieved October 22, 2008.
[114] McCann M, et. Al. *Enterolactone restricts the proliferation of the LNCaP human prostate cancer cell line in vitro.* Molecular Nutrition and Research, April 2008.
[115] Benson E, *In His Steps,* Ensign, September 1988, 2.
[116] www.whfoods.com. Retrieved October 22, 2008.
[117] Adam K, Liu R. *Antioxidant activity of grains.* Journal of Agriculture and Food Chemistry 2002; 50:6182-87.
[118] Hinckley G, *Come and Partake,* Ensign, May 1986, 49.
[119] Smith J, *Church History and Modern Revelation,* 1:383.
[120] Smith J, Improvement Era, February 1956, pp. 78-79.
[121] Merrill R, *Life expectancy among LDS and Non-LDS in Utah,* 2004. Retrieved November 11, 2008, from www.demographic-research.org/volumes/vol10/3/.
[122] Lyon J, Gardner K, Gress R, *Cancer incidence among mormons and non-mormons in Utah,* 1971. Retrieved November 4, 2008 from www.ncbi.nlm.nih.gov/pubmed/8167262.
[123] Murray, M, et al., *The condensed encyclopedia of healing foods,* Pocket Books Publishing, 2006.
[124] Haas E, Levin B, *Staying healthy with nutrition,* Celestial Arts Publishing, 2006.
[125] Haas E, Levin B, *Staying healthy with nutrition,* Celestial Arts Publishing, 2006.
[126] Mozian, L, *Foods that fight disease,* Avery Publishing, 2000.
[127] Shahidi, F, *Antinutrients and phytochemicals in food.* American Chemical Society 1997.